Men in Nursing

Chad E. O'Lynn, PhD, RN, is an instructor at the University of Portland School of Nursing. He earned his associate degree in nursing from Clackamas Community College in 1986; his bachelor of science degree in communication from Portland State University in 1984; his master's in nursing from Oregon Health & Science University in 1992; and his doctorate in health administration from Kennedy-Western University in 2003. He is currently a candidate for his doctorate in nursing from Oregon Health & Science University. He has served in leadership positions in the American Association of Neuroscience Nurses, and is currently on the board of directors of the American Assembly for Men in Nursing. He has published on topics including men in nursing, rural nursing, and neuroscience. His current research interests include gender issues in nursing, men in nursing, rural nursing, and men's health.

Russell E. Tranbarger, EdD, RN, FAAN, is professor emeritus at East Carolina University. He earned his diploma in nursing from the Alexian Brothers Hospital in Chicago in 1959; his bachelor of science degree in nursing from DePaul University in 1966; his master of science degree in nursing from the University of North Carolina at Chapel Hill in 1970; and his doctorate in education from North Carolina State University in 1991. He has published on topics including men in nursing, nursing informatics, and nursing leadership and administration. Dr. Tranbarger has held a number of faculty and hospital administration positions over the years and has served a variety of professional organizations, including the Council on Graduate Education in Administration of Nursing, the American Nurses Association, the North Carolina Foundation for Nursing, the North Carolina Institute of Medicine, and the North Carolina Board of Nursing. He recently completed two terms as president of the American Assembly for Men in Nursing and served six years as editor of *Interaction*. He is a fellow of the American Academy of Nursing.

Men in Nursing

*History, Challenges,
and Opportunities*

Edited by

Chad E. O'Lynn, PhD, RN

and

Russell E. Tranbarger, EdD, RN, FAAN

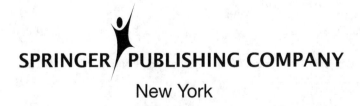

SPRINGER PUBLISHING COMPANY

New York

Springer Publishing Company, LLC
11 West 42nd Street
New York, NY 10036

Acquisitions Editor: Sally J. Barhydt
Managing Editor: Mary Ann McLaughlin
Production Editor: Emily Johnston
Cover design: Joanne E. Honigman
Composition: Apex Covantage

07   08   09   10/   5   4   3   2   1

Library of Congress Cataloging-in-Publication Data

Men in nursing : history, challenges, and opportunities / Chad E. O'Lynn and Russell E. Tranbarger, editors.
    p. ; cm.
  Includes bibliographical references and index.
  ISBN 0-8261-0221-2
1. Nursing. 2. Male nurses. I. O'Lynn, Chad E. II. Tranbarger, Russell E.
[DNLM: 1. Nurses, Male. 2. Nursing. 3. Prejudice.
  WY 191 M534 2006]
  RT41.M46 2006
  610.73081--dc22   2006018585

Printed in the United States of America by Bang Printing.

A dedication for the first book written about and for men in nursing requires the consideration of numerous people. Among them are L. Bissel Sanford, RN, the first man to become registered as a nurse in the United States; Leroy Craig and Brother Maurice Wilson, directors of schools of nursing for men, who advocated strongly for their students and graduates; and the many men who served in the military when their educational and nursing skills were ignored. However, one individual stands above the rest for his unending advocacy for men in nursing and for his vision in strengthening nursing as a profession: Luther Christman, PhD, RN, FAAN.

It is with humility then that we dedicate this book to Dr. Luther Christman. More than simply our attempt to honor him, it is our attempt to thank him for all he has done for his clients, for his beloved profession of nursing, and for his consistent promotion of men in nursing.

Chad E. O'Lynn and Russell E. Tranbarger

Contents

PART III. INTERNATIONAL PERSPECTIVES
Chad E. O'Lynn

PART IV. FUTURE DIRECTIONS
Russell E. Tranbarger

List of Tables

List of Figures

Contributors

Wally J. Bartfay, PhD, RN, is associate professor and coordinator (Nursing) in the Faculty of Health Sciences at the University of Ontario Institute of Technology. He earned his diploma in nursing sciences from Dawson College in 1985; his bachelor of arts degree in health sociology from McGill University in 1988; his bachelor of science degree in nursing from Brandon University in 1990; his master's in nursing from the University of Manitoba in 1993; and his doctorate from the University of Toronto in 1999. He has held a number of faculty positions in various schools of nursing in Manitoba and Ontario. His recent and current research interests include stroke, genetic disorders of iron metabolism, caregiver health, and cardiac and cardiovascular health.

William T. Bester, MSN, CRNA, is professor of clinical nursing at the University of Texas at Austin School of Nursing. He earned his bachelor of arts degree in nursing from the College of St. Scholastica in 1974; his certification as a registered nurse anesthetist from the U.S. Army School of Nurse Anesthesia in 1979; and his master of science degree in nursing from the Catholic University of America in 1985. He received honorary doctorates from the College of St. Scholastica in 2001 and from Seton Hall University in 2003. He served 30 years in the U.S. Army, rising to the rank of brigadier general, and served as chief of the Army Nurse Corps from 2000 to 2004. He served as the director of nursing for Project Hope's Tsunami Relief Health Care Team in 2005. He is the 2005 recipient of the American Assembly for Men in Nursing's Luther Christman Award.

Deborah A. Burton, PhD, RN, CNAA, is the regional director of nursing education and performance for Providence Health System, Portland, OR. She is also currently a member of the faculty at the University of Portland School of Nursing. She earned her bachelor of science degree in nursing from the University of Portland in 1977; her master's in nursing from Oregon Health and Science University in 1982; and her doctorate in nursing from Oregon Health and Science University in 1993. Her recent research and grant activities have focused on nurse recruitment, the recruitment of men into nursing, and nurse residency programs. She is currently providing consultancy services to several state-based nursing workforce centers.

Sara E. Hayden, PhD, is professor of communication studies at the University of Montana. She earned her bachelor of arts degree from the University of Wisconsin in 1987; her master of arts degree from the University of Minnesota in 1991; and her doctorate from the University of Minnesota in 1994. Her recent and current research interests include women and gender in communication, media, and rhetoric. She is currently the editor of *Women's Studies in Communication* and the associate editor of the *Western Journal of Communication*.

Brian J. Keogh, MScN, is a lecturer at the School of Nursing and Midwifery Studies at Trinity College, Dublin. He earned his bachelor of nursing studies degree from the University of Ulster at Jordanstown in 1998; his postgraduate diploma in further and higher education in 1999; his postgraduate diploma in education for nurses, midwives, and health visitors in 2002; his master of science degree in advanced nursing in 2002; and his postgraduate diploma in statistics in 2004. His recent and current research interests include eating disorders, gender in nursing, and nursing education.

Susan A. LaRocco, PhD, RN, is associate professor at the Curry College School of Nursing. She earned her bachelor of science degree in nursing from Boston College in 1976; her master of science degree in nursing from Boston University in 1977; her master of business administration degree from New York University in 1986; and her doctorate in nursing from the University of Massachusetts/Boston College of Nursing and Health Sciences in 2004. She currently serves on the board of directors of the American Assembly for Men in Nursing. Her recent research interests include nurse recruitment and men in nursing.

Terry R. Misener, PhD, RN, is dean of the University of Portland School of Nursing. He earned his bachelor of science degree in nursing from the University of Colorado in 1966; his master's degree in health science/family nurse practitioner from the University of California at Davis in 1973; and his doctorate in nursing science from the University of Illinois in 1981. He was the 2003 recipient of the American Assembly for Men in Nursing's Luther Christman Award. He has authored numerous publications and grants focusing on men's health, HIV/AIDS care, and graduate nursing education.

Daniel J. Pesut, PhD, APRN-BC, FAAN, is professor and chairperson of the Department of Environments for Health at the Indiana University/Purdue University Indianapolis School of Nursing. He is also the associate dean for graduate programs. He earned his bachelor of science degree in nursing from Northern Illinois University in 1975; his master of science degree in nursing from the University of Texas Health Science Center in 1977; his doctorate in nursing from the University of Michigan in 1984; and his postdoctorate in management development from Harvard University in 1999. He was the 2002 recipient of the American Assembly for Men in Nursing's Luther Christman Award. He served as president of Sigma Theta Tau International from 2003 to 2005, and is a fellow of the American Academy of Nursing. He has written extensively, including several nursing textbooks. His research interests include leadership, clinical reasoning, creative teaching and learning, environmental health, health services delivery, and health care administration.

Demetrius J. Porche, DNS, RN, FNP, CS, is professor and associate dean for nursing research and evaluation at the Louisiana State University Health Science Center School of Nursing. He earned his bachelor of science degree in nursing from Nicholls State University in 1987; his master's in nursing from Louisiana State University in 1989; his doctorate in nursing science from Louisiana State University in 1995; and his postmaster's certificate as a family nurse practitioner from Concordia University, WI, in 1999. He is a Virginia Henderson Fellow of Sigma Theta Tau International, and serves on the board of directors of the American Assembly for Men in Nursing. He has written extensively and has served as a consultant with governmental and community organizations. His recent research interests include nursing education, HIV/AIDS health and prevention, men's health, and community health.

Tim Porter-O'Grady, EdD, RN, CS, CNAA, FAAN, is a senior partner in Tim Porter-O'Grady Associates, Inc., and a senior consultant with Affiliated Dynamics, Inc., in Atlanta. He earned his bachelor of science degree in nursing from Seattle University in 1975; his master's in nursing administration from the University of Washington in 1977; and his doctorate in education from Nova-Southeastern University. He has earned postdoctoral certifications in advanced wound care, health care conflict resolution, mediation and arbitration, and gerontology. He is the chair of the board of directors of the Georgia Nurses Foundation and was the 2000 recipient of the American Assembly for Men in Nursing's Luther

Christman Award. He serves on the advisory board of the *Journal of Clinical Nursing* and has written extensively and authored or contributed to 13 books. Dr. Porter-O'Grady is a fellow of the American Academy of Nursing.

Larry D. Purnell, PhD, RN, FAAN, is professor at the University of Delaware College of Health and Nursing Sciences. He earned his bachelor of science degree in nursing from Kent State University in 1973; his master of science degree in nursing from Rush University in 1977; and his doctorate in health services administration from Columbia Pacific University in 1981. He recently served as a visiting professor/Fulbright Fellow at the Centre for Studies in Transcultural Health at Middlesex University in London, England. He has extensive consultation experience and has written extensively in the field of transcultural nursing. He is widely known for his Purnell Model of Cultural Competence. He has also published on emergency care, medical-surgical nursing, physiology, and health care management. He serves on a number of editorial boards of health-related journals and is a fellow of the American Academy of Nursing.

Eleanor J. Sullivan, PhD, RN, FAAN, is a nurse author, publishing novels as well as professional texts on nursing leadership, management, and substance abuse. She was formerly professor and dean of the University of Kansas School of Nursing. She earned her bachelor of science degree in nursing from St. Louis University in 1975; her master's in nursing from Southern Illinois University in 1977; and her doctorate in philosophy of education from St. Louis University in 1981. She served as president of Sigma Theta Tau International from 1997 to 1999 and as editor of the *Journal of Professional Nursing* from 1997 to 2002. She was the 2001 recipient of the American Assembly for Men in Nursing's Luther Christman Award. She is a fellow of the American Academy of Nursing. Dr. Sullivan is author of *Twice Dead* (Hilliard & Harris, 2002) and *Deadly Diversion* (Hilliard & Harris, 2004), mysteries that feature men in nursing.

Christina G. Yoshimura, PhD, is an adjunct assistant professor in the Department of Communication Studies at the University of Montana. She earned her bachelor of science degree in communications from Syracuse University in 1998; her master of arts degree in communications from Arizona State University in 2000; and her doctorate in communications from Arizona State University in 2004. She has recently taught a variety of courses on the topics of gender, family, and relational communications. Her current research interests include work/family conflict and communication in families. She is a member of the National Communication Association and the Western States Communication Association.

Preface

Nearly 25 years ago, I found myself at one of those crossroads in life. I was nearing the completion of a liberal arts bachelor's degree, and like so many graduating college students, I had no clue as to which career would utilize the education I had worked so hard to complete. I feared that I would be one of those proverbial waiters, waiting tables while waiting for something better to come along. While scanning the employment section in the local paper, I noticed the numerous employers seeking registered nurses. "Nursing?" I asked myself, "Why not?" I convinced myself that nursing wouldn't be so bad. After all, I would make more money than I would waiting tables, and if nursing was like what I'd seen on television, it would be easier work than waiting tables—that is, until a real career came along. Within a few weeks, I was enrolled in an associate's degree program at a local community college.

On the first day of class, I noted two other men in a class of about 30 nervous students. One of the men was a student from the Middle East who admitted that he was in nursing school only until he could get into medical school. He disappeared after a few weeks, possibly because he received an admission letter from a medical school, but more likely because he found the detailed lecture on how to fold a washcloth while providing a bedbath not to his liking. The other student was a recent immigrant from Samoa. He was a likable, good-humored fellow, but his struggles with the English language earned him a one-way ticket out of the program. For much of my program, I was the only male presence in the entire department.

My male sex separated me emphatically from the others. My classmates wore blue-and-white striped jumpers with starched white blouses and white hose. I wore some sort of polyester tunic that gave me the appearance of a crazed orderly from an old B movie. My classmates frequently discussed their boyfriends, or their husbands, or their experiences with childbirth and childrearing during lunch. I either sat silently or tried to change the topics of the conversations. My instructors spoke frequently about nursing traditions in a manner that made me think I had to genuflect at the mere mention of Florence Nightingale's name. I was never told that there were many men in nursing's past.

My gender isolation was overwhelming. I never saw a male registered nurse on any of the units where I had my clinical experiences; I certainly had no opportunity to work with one. At one hospital, I encountered male orderlies. I remember sitting in the break room one shift while the nurses commented on what "stupid clods" the orderlies were and how lazy they were, but thank God, they were strong and could move the patients for the nurses. As was typical in those times, I was forbidden to provide care on the postpartum unit, other than dumping laundry and measuring vital signs. If not for the unsanctioned actions of a staff nurse, I would never have been exposed to the labor and delivery unit. Of course, there were no men on the faculty. And since our nursing program had no interaction with other nursing programs, I was not aware of any other male students with whom I could connect for peer support.

My story of my experiences in nursing school is probably not very different from that of other men at the time. Clearly, I had many reasons to leave the program in anger, but I found the nursing courses challenging, and I felt that leaving would be admitting defeat to the insensitive treatment. I considered pursuing yet another degree, but I was broke and needed to work. I graduated, eventually, but with a heavy chip on my shoulder. Fortunately, I was hired by a hospital that placed me on a unit staffed by a number of former military nurses. These nurses seemed to have no issues with male nurses. There was too much work to be done to fuss about gender. These nurses became wonderful personal mentors, who made me quickly forget about my experiences in nursing school and, instead, made me focus on becoming the best nurse my talents would allow. Without these mentors, I would never have stayed in nursing.

Years later, my career took me to a faculty role in a baccalaureate nursing program. In 2000, I read a nursing article that happened to mention the American Assembly for Men in Nursing (AAMN). I had never heard of this organization and was immediately intrigued. I logged onto their Web site and found a discussion forum. I spent the afternoon reading previous postings. Many of the forum postings came from angry, frustrated, and isolated male nursing students. Their comments struck a visceral chord deep inside me, churning up long-forgotten memories of my own student experiences. Over the next week, I met with men enrolled in our nursing program. I was saddened to hear these students recount negative gender-based experiences. I was filled with disbelief, discovering that the same old stuff was going on right under my nose. I wondered if gender insensitivity was so insidious that even I didn't recognize it. After some reflection, I realized that I, along with the rest of the nursing profession, had been in denial. And at what cost was this denial? I wondered how common was the coping strategy expressed by one student, who said, "Yeah, it's there, but I just put up with it."

Several months later, I attended the annual conference of the AAMN. I spoke with numerous men of different ages, of different educational backgrounds, from different clinical areas, and from different parts of the country. I asked many of them about their gender experiences, and I was astounded by the similarity of the experiences these men shared. Many had considered leaving nursing at some point, in part because of these gender experiences. However, the love these men have for their clients and their work and their dedication to nursing have kept them in the ranks. During one of the conference sessions, a gentleman asked what could be done to help male nursing students. It was a rhetorical question of sorts. I observed many in the audience nodding their heads in recognition of the concern, but few offered any substantive comment. I left that conference determined to do something. First, I decided to learn more about the barriers men face in nursing school. What are they? How prevalent are they? How important are they? What can be done about them? My work in answering these questions is still underway, but initial progress has been made and is discussed in two chapters in this text. Second, in researching how to best answer these questions, I came across no book, out of all the books written about nursing, that focused on men. Consequently, I decided it was high time that a book should be published on men in nursing for men in nursing.

The foremost purpose of this book is to address the isolation men feel as nurses. Few nurses—men or women—have been taught anything about the historical role men have played in shaping the profession, and few men have received any acknowledgment of or support for the unique skills and talents that they bring to nursing. As a result, men may wonder about their relevancy in nursing. For men, and for the nursing profession as a whole, this book aims to articulate the barriers men face as nurses, the needs men have as nurses, strategies for change, and future opportunities for men in nursing. The book addresses these aims with reviews, personal biographies, and original research, organized into four sections.

Part I, Our History, focuses on the historical roles and contributions men have made to nursing over the centuries. Although a number of previous texts (usually written by women) have given brief mention to men's history in nursing, these texts have diminished men's contributions by implying that men were nurses only secondarily, with other roles, such as soldiers or members of the clergy, coming first. The chapters in this section aim to provide a more in-depth discussion of the work, compassion, and vision that men have contributed. It is hoped that this history will give men a sense of their place in nursing and also provide them with inspirational role models.

Part II, Current Issues, focuses on the challenges that men face in nursing today. The chapters in this section discuss how gender serves as a foundation for many of the obstacles, the discrimination, and the barriers experienced by men in nursing, as well as explaining the differences in communication and caring styles between male and female nurses. Importantly, the authors of these chapters also provide concrete recommendations to address these challenges. It is hoped that the chapters in Part II will not only assist men in overcoming barriers but will also help the nursing profession recognize and remove the often subtle and covert structural obstacles it places before men.

The chapters in Part III, International Perspectives, focus on men in nursing outside the United States. Despite sociocultural and historical differences, there are international similarities in the experiences of men in nursing. Readers outside the United States may take heart in knowing that their challenges are not unique and may find some of the recommendations provided in this book helpful in addressing issues in their own countries.

In Part IV, Future Directions, the reader is guided to look ahead. Readers may find this the thinnest section, and this observation may be justified. Men today are rewriting their nursing history and nursing realities. What the future holds for men in nursing is yet to be written. My expectation is that further texts will explicate our journey in shaping the nursing profession of the 21st century.

Perhaps in some ways, we have begun to turn a corner within the profession. Last summer, I received a letter from a gentleman who recounted a recent incident in which he and three male nurse colleagues were discussing with a female student the benefits of a nursing career. Sitting with these four men, the female student commented that large numbers of men were working on the hospital unit to which she was assigned. One of the men commented on her observation by telling her that studying to become a nurse was honorable, but that if she was ever given the opportunity to become a "male" nurse, she should pursue it (D. Drake, personal communication, July 2005). Humorous as it might be, this comment reveals the pride these men have as nurses. However, I fear that in too many environments, such pride is seldom seen.

It is hoped that men will find this book informative, inspirational, and a catalyst for the pride mentioned above. For me personally, a book such as this would have helped me find relevancy and vision as a male nursing student. Although this book would not have changed my immediate educational environment, it would have helped me articulate my struggles to those around me and advocate for possible change. Most importantly, this book would have established a connection with my male colleagues despite my solitary status in my individual nursing program.

In retrospect, a book such as this might well have lessened the size of the chip on my shoulder and would likely have instilled an even stronger motivation for me to stay in nursing. I hope this book will also inform our female nurse colleagues and move them to embrace a full recognition and appreciation of men in nursing. Nursing will only be strengthened if we proudly acknowledge our diversity and support each other as we move boldly into our shared future.

Chad E. O'Lynn

Foreword

For years I watched male colleagues in my profession exhibit skill, compassion, and professionalism as they filled positions in health care, in education, and in nursing associations. Could they, I wondered, experience types of discrimination similar to those that women faced in other arenas?

One Monday morning I invited all the male students in our nursing program to meet with me. I offered donuts. As I closed the door to the conference room, I told them that I didn't want to know their names, nor did I expect them to use names in recounting events. I only wanted them to talk freely about their academic experiences.

After a few minutes of uncomfortable silence, each of the 12 spoke glowingly about the program, how they loved nursing, were glad they'd enrolled, expected a great future, and so on. I asked if they had experienced any discrimination because they were men. Quickly they assured me they had not.

"Have more donuts," I offered.

Finally the stories emerged. One man spoke of missing the end-of-rotation celebration because his instructor sent him back to do another well-baby check. When he asked if he had made any mistakes, she said, "No. I just think you need to do another one."

Another man told how an instructor had repeatedly carried out postconferences when she and the female students were still in the locker room. When they emerged and he asked about the discussion, the instructor told him to ask one of the women.

This fine book, edited by Chad O'Lynn and Russell Tranbarger, explores a subject that has too long been taboo in nursing—equality for men in nursing. The authors included here will enlighten you, inform you, and help you understand men's experiences. They tell it like it is. And it will anger you that we remain so far from the ideal.

The rationale for women to be admitted to previously male-dominated professions posited that half of the world's talent was wasted when women were excluded. The same holds true for men in nursing. That so many men have had the fortitude to survive and often flourish in nursing is nothing less than remarkable.

There are numerous reasons for the lack of men in nursing. Originally deemed suitable only for the dregs of society (remember Dickens' Sairey Gamp?), the profession attracted few skilled nurses, men or women. Fortunately that changed, and for many years bright young women chose nursing as one of the three professions open to women. (Becoming a teacher or a secretary were the only other options.) More recently, affirmative action initiatives and persistence have ensured that women could enter professions previously closed to them; sadly, no such remedies have guaranteed men parity in nursing.

The media haven't helped. The portrayal of female nurses is often negative or at the very least inaccurate; men in nursing are simply absent, confirming the public's assumption that "real" men don't do nursing. Thus, the goal of recruiting more men into nursing has remained as elusive as ever; only the most enlightened and determined need apply.

At a time when all of the world's talent must be tapped to provide the top-notch quality of health care that we all need and deserve, no profession can afford to ignore any of its brightest and best. Gender neutrality in nursing must be attained; our future patients deserve it.

Thankfully, this book will help.

Eleanor J. Sullivan, PhD, RN, FAAN
Former Dean, University of Kansas School of Nursing
Past President, Sigma Theta Tau International

PART I

Our History

Over the years, many articles and books have reviewed the stories and events that have been significant to the nursing profession. Some of these publications have focused on a specific context or event, whereas others have provided a more comprehensive review of the development of the profession. The focus of each publication reflects the interests of the author, the publisher, and/or the anticipated audience. Since women have comprised the majority of nurses and nurse authors in modern times, these interests have been directed toward women. This has not been entirely bad. From a metaperspective, many general historians have neglected the historical contributions women have made to society. In this situation, the study of the history of nursing serves as one vehicle with which to study the history of women. Nursing serves as a visible example of the valuable contributions women have made, as well as revealing a vestige of the discriminatory gendered roles forced onto women.

However, previous publications have neglected to provide a full history of nursing. Many aspects of nursing's past remain largely unexplored, including the history of men in nursing. Part I of this book aims to provide the beginning of a journey into this historical territory. Although a truly exhaustive and international account of the history of men in nursing is not included here, part I does provide a more comprehensive account than has been found up to now in the nursing literature. The chapters in part I include information that has never before been published, such as an overview of the development of a nursing organization formed specifically to address the needs and concerns of men in nursing. The information provided in part I will help all nurses of today to more fully understand their collective past. Such an understanding is essential in addressing the challenges faced today by the nursing profession.

—Chad E. O'Lynn

CHAPTER ONE

History of Men in Nursing: A Review

Chad E. O'Lynn

INTRODUCTION

When a recent (2003) edition of Howard Zinn's history of the United States appeared, both praise and criticism erupted. What makes Zinn's history unique is that he presents historical events from the perspectives of minorities, the poor, and the dispossessed. The effects of historical events on these individuals have been overlooked by most historians, with the result that common historical knowledge is biased and limited. For example, few Americans learned in school that the expeditions of Christopher Columbus to North America resulted in appalling exploitation and genocide for indigenous peoples of the Caribbean. Interpretations of a shared history often differ among participants, as seen in the tension between the governments of China and Japan over the retelling of the story of the Japanese occupation of China during World War II.

There is a general misconception that historians are objective in revealing historical facts (Zinn, 2003). Yet history is rarely "objective," since events occur within a social, cultural, and political context. Zinn notes that

> By the time I began teaching and writing, I had no illusions about "objectivity," if that meant avoiding a point of view. I knew that a historian...was forced to choose, out of an infinite number of facts, what to present, what to omit. And that decision inevitably would reflect, whether consciously or not, the interests of the historian. (p. 683)

In many societies, historians come from the educated elite. As such, historians have represented the interests of the majority and of the powerful. Unfortunately, the solitary, limited voice of the historian can be passed down from generation to generation, resulting in the perpetuation of a skewed perspective on history.

And so it goes with nursing. Various authors have published historical reviews of the development of nursing as a profession. Since women comprise the majority of current nurses in most countries, and since most nurse historians have been female, most historical reviews represent the interests of women, even though men dominated nursing in earlier times (Bullough, 1994). This is evident in the overwhelming focus on female nurses in times when gender representation in nursing was far more balanced than it is today. It is also evident in the discounting of male nurses, by calling them attendants, assistants, or soldiers, or by giving little attention to them at all. For example, in discussing the role of men in the military nursing orders, Mellish (1990) states that "The main concern of the military nursing orders was the lives of the crusaders and not of the poor. Because of their military nature, there were no female members" (p. 44). This perspective is disproved by other authors (Donahue, 1996; Nutting & Dock, 1935; Sire, 1994). In another example of the dismissal of the role of men, in her large nursing text, Donahue (1996) devotes only one paragraph exclusively to men in nursing. A historical focus on women is especially evident in the choice of those who are held up as an inspiration for the profession. For example, Mellish identifies four female patron saints of nursing. However, the Catholic Church identifies eight patron saints of nursing, four of whom are male (Catholic Community Forum, 2002).

A major problem in reviewing the history of nursing is defining who was and who was not a nurse, particularly prior to the registration and/or licensure of nurses in modern times. Since the earliest times in human history, individuals have been singled out for their ability to tend to the injured and the sick. These healers, shamans, wise elders, and others utilized approaches and procedures consistent with current conceptualizations of nursing and medicine. Consequently, the history of nursing is closely intertwined with the history of medicine (Sapountzi-Krepia, 2004). However, at different times in different cultures, the roles of physician and nurse began to separate, so that physicians received specialized training and focused on evaluating patients and prescribing treatment. This pattern was solidified when the early European universities barred women from enrollment, thus allowing only men to be trained as physicians (Bullough & Bullough, 1993). On the other hand, nurses with varying lengths of apprenticeship became the renderers of care, spending larger amounts of time with patients than did physicians. As these roles of physicians and nurses became more distinct, authors have taken great liberties in identifying who was a nurse and in what settings nursing took place. For example, in her review of nursing in ancient Greece, Sapountzi-Krepia (2004) states that trained male nurses were actually physicians' assistants, and that the real nurses were the women of a patient's household. Theoretically, one could draw the same conclusion about today's hospital nurses. Similarly, in a response to a comment that men were the first nurses, Bainbridge (2001) argues that

> the suggestion that men were the first nurses is inherently sexist and ridiculous. It is based on the history of war in which women were ignored. Which begs the question, "While these male nurses were caring for men wounded in battle, who was caring for the women and children at home?" (p. 8)

Central to this question is whether or not a nurse must work outside the home to be considered a nurse. Using today's perspective, individuals who care for family members at home are considered parents or caregivers, whereas those caring for nonfamily members outside the home in exchange for financial reimbursement are more consistent with today's nurses. With the obvious exceptions of midwives and wet nurses, most societies agreed, if not mandated, that only men should work outside the home in a fashion consistent with today's nurse. After the establishment of the early Christian Church, the opportunities for women to partake in formal nursing expanded (Donahue, 1996). In later centuries, these opportunities were often provided only at the expense of joining a religious order. Men, on the other hand, had numerous opportunities for formal nursing, both inside and outside of religious orders, well into the 19th century.

Another problem in identifying who was or who was not a nurse centers on the fact that many individuals had multiple roles. In discussing the work of early nurses, authors frequently imply that men established hospitals and served as administrators or established religious orders for women, while leaving up to the reader's imagination the question as to who (presumably women) actually provided hands-on nursing care. At the same time, authors imply that deaconesses, widows, and Roman matrons not only established hospitals but diligently tended to the sick as well. Perhaps the clearest example of this problem is seen when discussing the members of the military nursing orders. Some authors (Bainbridge, 2001; Donahue, 1996; Mellish, 1990) describe these nurses as soldiers first, providing nursing care to the war wounded only out of necessity or out of boredom between military pursuits. Such a description implies rather inaccurately that these men should be identified only by a primary role. Such logic challenges the role identification of today's nurses who serve in the military, who are trained as soldiers and must take up arms when the need arises. One could argue that today's military nurses are nurses first, since the bulk of their time is spent nursing rather than soldiering. Using this logic, many of the men who served in the military nursing orders must be considered as nurses first, since the bulk of the nursing care was provided by low-ranking individuals, both monks and laymen, while high-ranking members of the military orders and knights conducted most of the soldiering (Bullough & Bullough, 1993; Nutting & Dock, 1935; Sire, 1994). Another example of the problem is seen in authors' descriptions of nursing during the American Civil War. Many soldiers were assigned to nurse the injured (Pokorny, 1992; Wilson, 1997). Many male civilians, such as Walt Whitman, provided nursing care as well (Kalisch & Kalisch, 2004; Wilson, 1997). However, these men have not been recognized for their work as nurses, even though Walt Whitman immortalized his nursing work in his poem "The Wound Dresser." On the other hand, female volunteers have been recognized for their nursing work with injured soldiers (Donahue, 1996; Kalisch & Kalisch, 2004; Nutting & Dock, 1935; Pokorny, 1992), even though military officers found these volunteers to be undisciplined and often motivated by curiosity (Kalisch & Kalisch, 1986, 2004).

Regardless of who was identified as a nurse and who was not, the fact remains that gendered societal roles and the sexual modesty inherent in many cultures led to health care being segregated between the sexes. Since nursing care often requires intimate contact with the patient, the nursing care of individuals outside the home setting was generally provided by nurses of the same sex as the patients until well into the 19th century. This sex-segregated nursing practice is still maintained in some Islamic societies. The transition to modern nursing, which became dominated by women in most countries, occurred prior to the transition to the social acceptability of trained women providing intimate care to men. As a result, the quality of the nursing care provided to many men began to plummet, generating calls for the recruitment and preparation of male nurses (Craig, 1940; Evans, 2004; Mackintosh, 1997).

The purpose of this chapter, then, is not to trivialize the importance of the contributions that women have made to the development of nursing and modern health care. Rather, the purpose is to provide the reader with a more comprehensive understanding of the history of the nursing profession. Although a detailed history of men in nursing is beyond the scope of this single chapter, the information on men in nursing provided here and in subsequent chapters in this book is much more comprehensive than is found in most reviews of the history of nursing. This chapter will serve as an adjunct to the reader's understanding of nursing history, much as Zinn's (2003) work serves as an adjunct to the common under-standing of American history. In particular, this chapter is significant for today's men in nursing, as men have not found role models or a sense of historical relevance in the nursing history that has previously been presented to them. This chapter will help counter the myths that men in nursing are a recent anomaly and that their inclusion is simply a move toward political correctness.

THE PRE-CHRISTIAN ERA

In ancient times, many individuals provided what would now be con-sidered nursing care to the sick. It is likely that this care was provided in the home, though we have few written records about this activ-ity or about those who provided this care. However, as the healing arts and sciences began to develop, so did the art and science of nurs-ing. The first known trained individuals to provide nursing care were men who were supervised by male physicians during the Hippocratic period of ancient Greece (Christman, 1988b; Davis & Bartfay, 2001). These early nurses were always male, due to society's restriction of women's roles to the home (Nutting & Dock, 1935; Sapountzi-Krepia, 2004). However, Sapountzi-Krepia (2004) suggests that these men only assisted the physician, and that ongoing nursing care was provided by the women of a household. It is not clear exactly what role these male assistants had in the provision of care. It is possible that they worked more like today's nurses in ambulatory care settings, rather than as extensions of a physician.

In ancient India, Hindus believed that the prevention of illness was more important than its cure (Nutting & Dock, 1935). As such, good hygiene and massage were considered to be vital for health. In the 3rd century B.C.E., King Asoka mandated that hospitals follow strict guidelines for cleanliness, ventilation, and comfort. The nurses working in these hospitals were almost always male (Nutting & Dock, 1935; Wilson, 1997). According to Lesson IX of the *Charkara-Samhita*, nurses should possess a knowledge of how drugs should be prepared and administered. In addition, nurses should be intelligent, loyal, and understand the relationships between the mind and the body. The first known formal school of nursing was started in India about 250 B.C.E. Only men were admitted to the school, as women were not considered "pure" enough to serve in this role (Wilson, 1997). Men were required to become skilled in cooking, bathing, and caring for patients, massage, physical therapy, and bedmaking, and they were required to be obedi-ent to the physicians (Nutting & Dock, 1935; Wilson, 1997). A later text of ancient Indian medicine, *Astangahrdayam*, was written probably sometime between 550 and 600 C.E. by an unknown author, but was attributed to the grandson of Vagbhata, a renowned physician (Murthy, 1994). In this text, Vagbhata notes, "The attendant (nurse) should be attached (affectionate, faithful to the patient), clean (in body, mind and speech), efficient in work and intelligent" (Murthy, 1994, p. 15). These requirements for ancient Indian nurses are not very different from those for nurses well into the 19th century.

In ancient Rome, the best nursing care was provided to soldiers. Initially, wounded soldiers were cared for in tents or private buildings by old men or women. However, military hospitals, known as *valetudinaria*, were established and male nurses, *nosocomi*, were employed in them (Nutting & Dock, 1935). These military hospitals continued to function until the fall of the Roman Empire.

THE EARLY CHRISTIAN ERA

Throughout the early Christian Era, the poor and sick flocked to the homes of bishops and other church officials in hope of receiving charity and care (Nutting & Dock, 1935). Provision of charity and care to the sick and poor was an important mission for many congregations, consistent with the teachings of Christ. As the numbers of the infirm arriving at churches swelled, many bishops added separate wings and cloisters to house them and meet their need for hospitality. Initially, members of the local congregation cared for these individuals under the direction of deacons and deaconesses. Thus, the original Christian hospitals were born. In time, congregation members were replaced by monks and nuns who served as nurses (Nutting & Dock, 1935). During the reign of Roman Emperor Justinian (527–565 C.E.), bishops were given authority over all hospitals, and soon the number of hospitals and shelters increased dramatically in the empire, as did the number of religious orders founded to care for the sick and the poor. Two individual men, Ephrem and Basil, who were later canonized as saints, are still recognized for their work in establishing nursing care for the infirm.

St. Ephrem served as a deacon in Edessa (located in present-day Turkey) in 350 C.E. at the time of a serious plague. Ephrem collected money from rich citizens in the town and bought 300 beds, which he installed in public porticoes and galleries to care for the sick. Ephrem visited the sick daily and cared for many of them with his own hands (Nutting & Dock, 1935). In 370 C.E., St. Basil the Great became the bishop of Caesarea (also located in present-day Turkey), which at the time was one of the major patriarchal sees in the Church (Knight, 2005e). Basil showed great interest in the care of the poor and the sick and often rebuked the rich and privileged for their lack of Christian charity. In response to the opulent homes of the rich, he used the Church's resources to build a magnificent collection of buildings in the suburbs. This small city next to Caesarea was known as Ptochoptopheion, or "Newtown," and contained quarters for the housing of travelers, for the care of the sick, and for the industrial training of the unskilled (Knight, 2005e). Also among these buildings was a ward for lepers. The care and compassion provided to lepers was so excellent that Newtown became known as the premier hospital for lepers. The hospital of Newtown became the flagship hospital of the Church at that time, and soon other hospitals in Constantinople and Alexandria were built using it as a model (Knight, 2005e; Nutting & Dock, 1935).

St. Basil employed a number of workers to care for the infirm, including male nurses (*nosocomi*) and men who sought out the sick and brought them to the hospital. The latter groups of men, known as *parabolani*, were used in a number of large cities throughout the empire. It is possible that these men also provided nursing care, akin to employees of a modern home health agency, in addition to their transport services. The *parabolani* provided an important service, particularly during the numerous plagues that periodically ravaged Europe and the Middle East, and authors have praised the work of these men (Donahue, 1996; Gomez, 1994; Mellish, 1990; Wilson, 1997). However, Nutting and Dock (1935) provide a more measured discussion of the *parabolani*. Nutting and Dock note that since the nature of illness was poorly understood, the work of these men was seen as undesirable and dangerous. As a result, the parabolani were composed of low-level monks and laymen who were pressed into service. In many cities, the *parabolani* became notorious for their brutish behavior, their illegal activities, and the taking of bribes in exchange for care. Nutting and Dock note that the activities of the *parabolani* became so bad that most bishops disbanded these groups by the middle of the 5th century.

The establishment of institutions to care for the sick and infirm flourished during the Byzantine period (324–1453 c.e.), particularly in the eastern Mediterranean region (Lascaratos, Kalantzis, & Poulakou-Rebelakou, 2004). Much of the impetus for creating such institutions stemmed from the Christian belief in charity that transformed the ethics and social structure in most Mediterranean cultures after the Roman capital was moved to Constantinople in the 4th century. Of particular note were the large numbers of facilities that cared for the aged, called *gerocomeia* (Greek for "elderly care"). Many of these ancient nursing homes were founded by emperors,

noblemen, and families of the gentry, and they were often built next
to established monasteries. One of the most important of these *gerocomeia* was located at the monastery and hospital of the Pantocrator
in Constantinople, established during the reign of Emperor John II
Comnenus (1118–1143) (Lascaratos et al., 2004). This *gerocomeia*
was designed to care for 24 patients under the care of six male nurses.
If a patient grew ill, a physician was notified, and the patient was
transferred to the hospital proper.

As the number of Byzantine hospitals grew, laypeople working as
paid nurses increasingly took over nursing care from monks and nuns,
a process that was nearly complete by the 6th century (Bullough &
Bullough, 1993). In this way, nursing became a separate and specialized
occupation. Most of these paid nurses were men, though in consistency
with the sex segregation of the times, women continued to staff the wom-
en's wards of Byzantine hospitals. However, the 13th-century hospital
for women at the Lips Monastery was staffed entirely by male nurses
(Bullough & Bullough, 1993). Female midwives continued to serve as
primary care providers for women during this era, both in the hospital
and in the home setting. Some midwives gained enough knowledge to
serve as both physicians and nurse healers for women in times of illness
(Bullough & Bullough, 1993).

Nurses, both male and female, were eligible to join guilds in
Byzantine cities, and, thus, earn a wage. Female and male nurses at the
Pantokrator hospital in Constantinople earned the same wage, and
may have even belonged to the same guilds (Bullough & Bullough,
1993). Guild membership required some formalized training, most
likely apprenticeship training, in nursing and professionalism,
although little is known about the content of nurses' education. The
use of such educated laypeople as nurses was not imitated in hospitals
in the western Mediterranean region, which continued to use men and
women affiliated with religious orders as nurses. The use of religious
as nurses may also have discouraged the formation of nursing guilds
in the western Mediterranean.

The pattern of establishing hospitals near religious institutions was
prevalent in early England as well as elsewhere. Nutting and Dock (1935)
cite Gasquet, who notes that the earliest English hospitals were infirma-
ries located next to a church or abbey. A male infirmarian was appointed
and required to

> have qualities similar to those that we are familiar with in the char-
> acterization of the ideal nurse. He should have the virtue of patience
> in a pre-eminent degree. He must be gentle and good-tempered, kind,
> compassionate to the sick, and willing, as far as possible, to gratify
> their needs with affective sympathy. (pp. 442–443)

THE MILITARY NURSING ORDERS

As mentioned earlier, the authors of some reviews of the history of nursing have suggested erroneously that only a minimal nursing contribution was made by members of military orders, or that nursing care focused primarily on the treatment of wounded soldiers. In addition, the usually brief mention of military nursing orders by authors does not inform the reader that activities and directions differed and changed among the orders over time. Some orders dropped their nursing focus over time, whereas other orders dropped their military focus over time. Hence, one cannot paint all the orders with the same brush. Four military nursing orders have received the most attention in previous reviews: the Knights Hospitallers of St. John of Jerusalem (now the Sovereign Military Order of Malta), the Knights of St. Lazarus, the Templar Knights, and the Teutonic Knights. These orders must be discussed within the context of the Crusades (Nutting & Dock, 1935); however, a full historical and political discussion of the Crusades and the Catholic Church is beyond the scope of this chapter.

Early hostels sheltered, fed, and most likely nursed sick Christian pilgrims coming to the Holy Land. These hostels began to appear as early as 603 c.e., when Pope Gregory the Great founded a hostel in Jerusalem (Sire, 1994). Initially, the governments of the Holy Land welcomed the pilgrims and the commerce they brought. Over the centuries, the ability of pilgrims to safely visit the Holy Land fluctuated with the political and military struggles in the eastern Mediterranean region. Near the conclusion of the first millennium, it was not uncommon for pilgrims to be robbed while on their travels or to be required to render bribes to local officials or thugs in order to gain access to holy sites (Nutting & Dock, 1935). Around the year 1050, the caliph of Egypt ruled over Jerusalem and gave wealthy merchants from the Italian city of Amalfi permission to build a compound with hospitals, a convent and monastery, and a church in Jerusalem (Bullough & Bullough, 1993; Nutting & Dock, 1935; Sire, 1994; Sovereign Order of Malta, 2005). One hospital, St. Mary Magdalene, was built to care for women, while another, St. John, was built to care for men (Nutting & Dock, 1935). Some historians believe that the men's hospital was named for St. John the Almsgiver, but since the abbey was built on the spot believed to be where an angel announced the conception of St. John the Baptist, it was St. John the Baptist who was the patron saint of this hospital and, later, the patron saint of the Knights Hospitallers of St. John of Jerusalem (subsequently referred to here as the "Hospitallers") (Sire, 1994). By 1080, the hospitals had become well known for the care provided to poor and sick pilgrims. The hospital servants who provided the nursing care were composed of the members of a lay fraternity associated with the monastery located at this site. It is presumed that women from an associated convent cared for the clients of St. Mary Magdalene (Bullough & Bullough, 1993). Bullough and Bullough contend that women played a minor role in nursing in medieval hospitals overall, though not in the home setting, since the founding of convents and female religious orders did not become commonplace until the 17th century. As such, it is likely that fewer hospitalized patients were women. The care provided at the Jerusalem hospitals was of such high quality that many pilgrims stayed behind to join the lay brothers and sisters in caring for the sick (Nutting & Dock, 1935).

At the time of the millennium, many Christians believed that the apocalypse was close at hand (Nutting & Dock, 1935). This belief spawned a sharp increase in the number of pilgrims traveling to the Holy Land and a sharp increase in crimes committed against them. Also, at this time, there was much infighting among European kingdoms and nobles. Due to these reasons, as well as other religious and political factors, Pope Urban II organized the First Crusade during the closing years of the 11th century. During the battles, many soldiers were cared for by the Hospitallers at their hospital. Upon the conquest of Jerusalem in 1099, Godfrey de Bouillon was so impressed with the Hospitallers that he granted them parcels of the newly conquered lands (Sire, 1994). Other noblemen followed suit, and soon the Hospitallers had great wealth. Under the supervision of the Hospitallers' leader, Brother Gerard, this newly acquired wealth was used to expand their hospital mission. In less than 15 years, seven other hospitals were built in Mediterranean ports (Sire, 1994). With the Holy Land now in Christian European hands, the number of pilgrims increased sharply. The new hospitals swelled with clients and, in gratitude for the care they received, payments to the Hospitallers swelled as well. Brother Gerard and his followers continued to expand their mission, building hospitals in Europe and a new, larger hospital to replace the two smaller hospitals in Jerusalem (Nutting & Dock, 1935; Sire, 1994).

Up to this point, the military role of the Hospitallers had not yet developed (Sire, 1994). The order was unique for the time in that it allowed men to follow a religious vocation yet still be active in the world. In other words, the men were not cloistered in the monastery. The intent at that time was to "form a group of lay brethren whose service to God was to be expressed less in corporate prayer than in active works of mercy" (Sire, 1994, p. 209). The lay brothers consisted primarily of former soldiers who had given up their arms to take vows of obedience, chastity, and charity. However, it is likely that Brother Gerard had some lay brothers keep their arms, assigning them to escort pilgrims landing on the coast and traveling the still dangerous roads to Jerusalem (Sire,

1994). By 1113, the number of Hospitallers had grown so large that Brother Gerard asked for the incorporation of the order under the auspices of the Vatican. This incorporation was granted on February 15, 1113, by Pope Paschal II (Sire, 1994; Sovereign Order of Malta, 2005), thus changing the Hospitallers from a secular order to a religious order, though it retained its authority to elect its own officials without Vatican interference. The Hospitallers adopted a white, eight-pointed cross as their symbol in honor of the eight beatitudes (Nutting & Dock, 1935; Sovereign Order of Malta, 2005).

In the Hospitallers' hospitals, the care provided was of a quality that had not been seen in other hospitals (Bullough & Bullough, 1993; Sire, 1994). When sick people arrived at one of the Hospitallers' hospitals, they were bathed and dressed in a clean gown and given a cloak and boots for coming in and out of the hospital. Clients were given their own bed, which was roughly square in shape to allow maximum comfort. Clients were to be fed and clothed before the brothers themselves were allowed to eat. Clients were fed fresh meat three times a week, something only the very wealthy could expect in the 12th century. In later years, clients were fed from silver bowls and spoons, in order to demonstrate the lavishness deserved by the sick (Sire, 1994). In the 12th century, the Jerusalem hospital housed and fed up to 2,000 guests, though not all guests were ill. Four physicians were assigned to the hospital, and nine brothers were assigned to each aisle of clients. The Jerusalem hospital became the model used by the famous Maisons-Dieu hospitals of France (Sire, 1994). It should be noted that the Hospitallers provided care not only for Christians but also for Muslim soldiers and citizens (Nutting & Dock, 1935; Sire, 1994).

In 1118, Raymond du Puy became the second leader of the Hospitallers, and it was on his watch that the order took on a military role (Nutting & Dock, 1935; Sire, 1994). After the death of Brother Gerard in 1120, some Hospitallers were relieved of escort duty and assigned to direct soldiering activities. At about the same time as Raymond was leader of the Hospitallers, another military nursing order, the Templar Knights, had established a hospital near the Temple of Solomon in Jerusalem (Sire, 1994). The Templars recruited European knights to come to Jerusalem to fight battles during the day and nurse the wounded at night. Hence, from the beginning, the Templars devoted a large amount of attention to military pursuits. It is possible that the Templars received a great deal of adulation for their military victories, which may have influenced Raymond to shift the Hospitallers into more aggressive military pursuits (Sire, 1994). Exactly how the Hospitallers reorganized themselves at this point is unclear, but it is likely that the Hospitallers who pursued military action did not take full religious vows, and those who did take such vows primarily busied themselves with nursing and religious pursuits. The distinction in terms of roles among individual Hospitallers remained murky until 1216 (Sire, 1994). By this time, there were three types of Hospitallers: knights, chaplains, and serving brothers. Knights were of patrician birth and served as leaders and soldiers. However, between battles, their work was to be devoted to the hospitals and the order. Chaplains were priests who ministered to the religious needs of the members and of clients. Serving brothers provided the bulk of the direct nursing care and hospitality services (Nutting & Dock, 1935; Sire, 1994). This three-tiered membership persisted in the order until the 16th century.

A similar membership structure was adopted by the Teutonic Knights. This order had its origins in a hospital established in Jerusalem about 1130 by a wealthy German merchant in order to serve German pilgrims to the Holy Land. The merchant's wife founded an adjoining hospital to serve female pilgrims (Nutting & Dock, 1935). The order was recognized by Pope Clement III in 1191, and it soon adopted the nursing practices of the Hospitallers. The Teutonic Knights developed collaborative relationships with the Hospitallers and the Templars, joining both in battles over the next few centuries (Opsahl, 1996). Although much of their history is documented in terms of their military pursuits, the order's "Book of the Order," written in 1264, states that a hospital must operate wherever the knights were headquartered (Sterns, 1969). The hospitals operated by the Teutonic Knights required that clients confess their sins prior to admission. Thus, it is highly unlikely that non-Christians were welcomed. Evans (2004), in paraphrasing the "Book of the Order," inaccurately determines that only women performed nursing duties in these hospitals. In reality, Sterns (1969) notes, the rules stated that *some* of the nursing duties were more appropriate for women to perform (most likely, those services rendered to female clients). Earlier in the book is a detailed listing of the nursing activities and responsibilities of the brethren. In subsequent centuries, the Teutonic Knights continued their military pursuits, involving themselves in conflicts with European powers and with the Hospitallers. The order was finally defeated and bankrupted in 1410 (Opsahl, 1996).

Throughout the 12th and 13th centuries, battles continued in the Holy Land. At times, alliances were struck among the Hospitallers, the Templars, and the Teutonic Knights; however, quarrels and political infighting for resources and dominance ultimately divided the orders, which assisted in the recapture of the Holy Land by surrounding Muslim nations (Sire, 1994). The Hospitallers lost control of Jerusalem in 1188, though the victorious Muslim army led by Saladin allowed the hospital to remain there for 12 months before being evacuated, in order to allow the sick to heal. The Hospitallers returned to Jerusalem in 1229, when

Frederick II took the city, but they were finally expelled from Jerusalem in 1244. The Hospitallers, along with the other knightly nursing orders, fled to other hospitals and bases outside Jerusalem, but they were defeated for the last time in the Holy Land when Acre fell in 1291 (Sire, 1994; Sovereign Order of Malta, 2005).

Initially, the Hospitallers fled to Cyprus, but in 1310 they settled in Rhodes. They continued building and staffing hospitals, but since the Christian world required a navy to defend itself against further expansion of Muslim-held territory, the Hospitallers also built and operated a fleet of Navy ships (Sovereign Order of Malta, 2005). The Hospitallers remained in Rhodes for some 200 years as a sovereign military power, continuing its mission to care for the sick and poor. In 1523, the Hospitallers lost the island of Rhodes to the Turks, but they were given the island of Malta in 1530 by Emperor Charles V with the blessing of Pope Clement VII. The condition for receipt of the island was that the Hospitallers would not raise arms against any Christian nation (Sovereign Order of Malta, 2005).

With the order's move to Malta, the Hospitallers lost much of their military power and subsequently pursued their nursing mission with vigor. When they arrived, the local Maltese population was already served by a hospital, so the Hospitallers built, for the first time in their history, a hospital for men only, which cared for wounded soldiers and sailors (Sire, 1994). Hospitals operated elsewhere by the Hospitallers continued to serve both men and women. As before, the Hospitallers continued to raise the bar for the quality of hospital care. By the 17th century, three physicians, one of which had to be a surgeon, were required to sleep at the hospital so as to be available day or night. In addition, all initiates into the order were required to work side by side with the nursing brothers once a week (Sire, 1994).

During this time, some of the knights of the Hospitallers attracted attention due to their compassion and devotion to the sick. For example, after a great deal of work converting the Huguenots in France to Catholicism, Gaspard de Simiane la Coste devoted himself to caring for the sick in prisons and in hospitals (Sire, 1994). He organized a mission to care for sick galley slaves in 1643, and later he established a hospital in Marseilles for them. He not only provided hands-on nursing care to these slaves but also lived at the hospital to be closer to them. His choice of residence likely proved fatal, as he died from the plague in 1649. Other Hospitallers responded to natural disasters, such as the earthquake in Messina, Italy, in 1783, with soup kitchens and field hospitals (Sire, 1994).

The Hospitallers were stripped of their riches during the French Revolution, and they were eventually removed from Malta by Napoleon's army in 1798 (Sire, 1994; Sovereign Order of Malta, 2005). Although the British retook Malta in 1800, the Hospitallers were not allowed to return. They eventually settled in Rome, giving up all military pursuits, though retaining the order's independence. The Hospitallers nearly ceased to exist in the years leading up to World War I. However, since the 1940s, the Hospitallers have become revitalized, operating a number of hospitals and ambulance services throughout Europe. In addition, the Hospitallers (now known as the Sovereign Order of Malta, or the Knights of Malta) have responded to international relief efforts, either independently or in conjunction with other relief organizations, such as AmeriCares (AmeriCares, 2003; Sire, 1994; Sovereign Order of Malta, 2005). The Knights of Malta is the only one of the original military nursing orders still in existence, with an almost 1,000-year tradition of tending to the needs of the sick and poor.

Perhaps the oldest of the military nursing orders is the Order of St. Lazarus of Jerusalem (Knights of St. Lazarus) (Nutting & Dock, 1935). The order traces its origins to the leper hospitals founded in the 4th century by St. Basil, but these origins are questionable, since the hospital founded in Jerusalem followed the religious traditions of the West, and not those of the East (Knight, 2005b). The order's hospital in Jerusalem focused on care for lepers. Unlike the clients of the other Jerusalem hospitals, who returned home after receiving care, lepers were not allowed to return to society. Thus, the clients of the leper hospital became inmates. The clients ultimately took religious vows and cared for each other (Knight, 2005b). Less is written about their hospital than about others, presumably because it had few visitors.

It is not clear when the Order of St. Lazarus took up arms like the other military nursing orders, but upon the fall of Acre in 1291, its members abandoned their hospital mission and devoted themselves to military pursuits until their assets were transferred to the Hospitallers in 1490 by Pope Innocent VIII. However, the Hospitallers took possession of the order's assets only in Germany, and the order continued with military pursuits. In 1567, Pope Pius V attempted to return the order to its original mission of caring for lepers, but leprosy was on the decline in Europe, and the return to nursing never took hold. The order ceased to exist during the turmoil surrounding the French Revolution (Knight, 2005b).

THE NONMILITARY NURSING ORDERS

A number of male nursing orders that never took up military arms flourished during the Middle Ages and the Renaissance in Europe. Unfortunately, these orders receive relatively little recognition in reviews of nursing history. One of these orders was the Brothers of St. Anthony. This order was founded by Gaston of Dauphine and his son in about the year 1095 (Evans, 2004; Knight, 2005c), in thanksgiving for a miraculous recovery from erysipelas, a bacterial cellulitis of the skin commonly known as St. Anthony's Fire. They built a hospital near the Church of St. Anthony at Saint-Didier de la Mothe, which specialized in treating this disorder. Initially, the brothers were laymen, but later, in the 13th century, they took monastic vows. The order established a number of hospitals throughout France, Spain, and Italy, and even had the privilege of caring for the sick in the papal household. In 1777, they merged with the Knights of Malta, but they disappeared after the French Revolution (Knight, 2005c).

Around 1180, Guy de Montpellier, a nobleman in France, established a hospital dedicated to the Holy Spirit. The hospital was staffed by laymen, and contrary to the custom of locating hospitals outside a city and away from people, Guy de Montpellier located his hospital in the center of town. The Brotherhood of Santo Spirito grew, and in 1204, Pope Innocent III summoned Guy de Montpellier to Rome to build a new hospital on the site of an old hospital, established in 715 by an Anglo-Saxon king, that had fallen into disrepair. The brothers, though laymen, were given privileges usually only given to members of the great monastic orders. Soon, the brotherhood grew, establishing hospitals across Europe. In return for the brothers' care, the brotherhood received gifts of land and riches, emboldening the brothers to consider adopting the practices of the military orders. This was halted by Pope Pius II. In 1476, Pope Sixtus IV decreed that the leadership of the brotherhood could be granted only to members of the clergy. Thus, the brothers never bore arms, and they continued with their charitable work of caring for the sick. It is believed that there were as many as 900 hospitals operated by the brotherhood across Europe (Knight, 2005d; Nutting & Dock, 1935).

Another order, the Alexian Brothers, started less formally, following the tradition of groups of celibate laymen and laywomen known as *béguines*, who cared for the sick and dying as early as the 12th century. By the middle of the 13th century, a group of men living along the Rhine became organized and dedicated themselves to caring for the sick. When the Black Death struck Europe in 1346, many families abandoned their sick relatives out of fear. The brothers stayed behind to care for the stricken and to bury the dead. After the plague, the group dedicated itself to St. Alexius, and soon the brotherhood became known as the Alexian Brothers. In 1472, the Alexian Brothers became a religious community and their numbers spread. In 1656, they rebuilt their hospital in Aachen, Germany, which had been destroyed by a fire. The new hospital was one of the first hospitals to specialize in the treatment of the mentally ill. During the French Revolution, most religious orders were abolished by law. The number of brothers declined to near zero, and the brotherhood was in danger of extinction. However, in 1856, Brother Dominic Brock began to rebuild the German community, and he was able to send brothers to care for the injured in the battlefields and field hospitals. The brotherhood grew exponentially, and soon hospitals and service to the sick spread to England, Ireland, and then the United States. The brothers provide nursing care for the sick to this day (Alexian Brothers, 2005).

Yet another order is the Hospitaller Brothers of St. John of God. This order was founded by Juan Ciudad, who was born in Portugal in 1495 (Knight, 2005a, 2005f). He spent his young adult life as a wanderer, engaging in military pursuits, farm labor, and the selling of religious books and cards. He traveled to Granada, Spain, after receiving a vision. There he was so inspired by the preaching of John of Avila that he gave away all his possessions and wandered the streets, banging his chest and asking God for mercy. He was committed to a psychiatric facility where his confessor instructed him to find a different way to atone for his sins. He decided to dedicate himself to the care of the sick and the poor and walked the streets of Granada searching for people to care for in his rented home. He even bore the afflicted on his shoulders if they could not walk. For some time, he was a one-man operation, begging for supplies at night and caring for the sick in his home during the day. He inspired two wealthy, local celebrities in Granada to join his operation, and together they formed the core of a growing congregation of men. Juan Ciudad died in Granada in 1550 while trying to save a drowning boy. He was canonized as St. John of God in 1690. The order grew after his death, and today the Hospitaller Brothers of St. John of God operate over 250 specialized hospitals and health centers in 49 countries (Hospitaller Brothers of St. John of God, 2005; Knight, 2005a, 2005f).

St. Camillus de Lellis is credited with founding another nursing order. Camillus was born in Italy in 1550 (Goodier, 1959). As a young man, Camillus was a troublemaker, addicted to gambling and making a living as a mercenary. After several attempts at turning his life around, he was finally accepted into a Franciscan monastery. However, Camillus suffered from a nonhealing leg wound that had persisted for years. He was told that he could not take vows with such an impediment, so he traveled to S. Giacomo hospital in Rome. There, he offered up his servitude in exchange for treatment for his wound. He worked as a nurse for four years while receiving spiritual guidance from St. Phillip Neri. St. Phillip Neri was so moved by Camillus that he made him superintendent of all the nurses, who at that time were all men. Camillus soon found that hard work kept his mind off his past temptations and motivated him to see his nursing work in a new light. Goodier notes that

> He began to love the patients in the hospital, not merely to serve them; and the more he loved them, the more he was troubled by the treatment they received, even in a well-regulated hospital like S. Giacomo. One evening...the thought occurred to him that good nursing depended on love and [how much better it would be] independent of wages. If he could gather men about him who would nurse for love, and leave the wages to look after themselves, then he might hope to raise nursing to the standard he desired. (para. 36)

Over the next few years, Camillus pursued this dream, first becoming ordained as a priest and then founding an order in the most pestilent neighborhood in Rome. Camillus noted that frequently, the sick were too debilitated to travel to the hospital. At that time, the dying were often left on their own, especially among the poor. Camillus realized that the sick outside the hospital were in more need of nursing care than those inside the hospital. He founded his congregation in 1586 to include a special devotion to comforting the dying, thus becoming the first home hospice of sorts. He and his followers became known for their charity and were soon called the Brothers of a Happy Death (also known as the Fathers of a Good Death, the Regulars of the Sick, or the Camillians). On his travels, Camillus carried coins in a purse for beggars along the road. Imitating the Good Samaritan, Camillus would carry the sick to the nearest inn and pay the innkeeper to provide nursing care. Camillus and his followers visited prisons, personally shaving and washing convicts and nursing those condemned to death (Goodier, 1959).

When the congregation was elevated to the rank of an order in 1591, the pope approved Camillus's request that the group be allowed to use a red cross as its symbol. Camillus served as leader of the order until his health began to fail in 1607. However, his poor health did not deter him from his nursing. He was known to drag himself to hospitals to nurse the sick, and when he was too ill to leave his house, he accepted the sick into his own bed. He died in 1614, but he is credited with the founding of the nursing spirit and the creation of the Red Cross symbol for the provision of humanitarian care to anyone seeking care (Goodier, 1959).

THE DARK AGES OF NURSING: THE DISAPPEARANCE OF MEN FROM NURSING?

Mellish (1990) refers to the years between 1500 and 1800 as the Dark Ages for nursing, although one could argue that this period extended until the reforms in nursing ushered in by Florence Nightingale in the second half of the 19th century. Unlike the field of medicine, which benefited from scientific advances during this period, nursing experienced a decline in its knowledge base, values, and status in many Western locales. A primary reason for this decline was the massive closure of monasteries and convents due to the upheavals of the Protestant Reformation. Prior to the Reformation, most hospitals were staffed and managed by various religious orders. When monks and nuns were driven out of northern European countries, they took their nursing knowledge and literature with them (Donahue, 1996). As a result, many hospitals were turned over to secular organizations that lacked the discipline to keep hospitals orderly and often employed untrained nurses of questionable character (Donahue, 1996; Kalisch & Kalisch, 2004; Mellish, 1990). With the drop in the number of hospitals run by religious orders, written accounts of men in nursing and their experiences also began to decline.

The number of men in religious orders devoted to nursing declined for other reasons as well. The period between 1500 and 1800 saw an increase in the number of women entering religious life in Catholic countries, and these women were often directed toward hospital service. Although men continued to work as nurses when intimate care for men was needed or when physical strength was required to subdue confused or mentally ill patients (Evans, 2004; Mackintosh, 1997), larger numbers of hospitals, such as the Maisons-Dieu of France, requested nuns as nurses (Nutting & Dock, 1935). Also, some of the male nursing orders ceased to exist due to disruptions in donor support from an increasingly fragile nobility, political infighting, military pursuits, and outright banning of activities by governments such as that of the French Revolution and Napoleonic France (Alexian Brothers, 2005; Knight, 2005b, 2005c).

Within the context of war, men continued to nurse the injured in battlefield hospitals throughout this period. Men also continued to work as nurses in contexts where female nurses were nonexistent or in short supply, as in the exploration and colonization of the Americas. Wilson (1997) notes that the first self-identified European nurse to set foot in what is now the United States was Friar Juan de Mena. Friar Juan de Mena had a long career of nursing in Mexico, though he never practiced on American soil. He was shipwrecked off the Texas coast and was soon killed by Indians. In Canada, the first known European nurses were Jesuit missionaries and male attendants at the French settlement at Port Royal, Acadia (Davis & Bartfay, 2001). Also during this period, James Derham, a black slave, earned enough money working as a nurse to purchase his freedom in 1783 (Carnegie, 1995). Derham eventually moved to Philadelphia and became a renowned physician.

Another context in which men worked as nurses but have received little attention was the periodic epidemics that swept the American South in the 19th century (Sabin, 1997). In this highly segregated and patriarchal society, White men were expected to be protectors and leaders of their families and White communities. Outbreaks of yellow fever, typhoid, smallpox, dengue fever, and the like ravaged Southern communities, causing many healthy residents to flee. Chivalrous men were expected to send their female family members and children elsewhere, while they stayed behind to nurse the sick, keep order, and protect assets. In addition, many African American men not allowed to flee served as nurses for White residents, as well as for those in their own communities. Many men served tirelessly, tending the sick for days on end. Sabin (1997) notes that men served in two different roles: one the role of a domestic or private-duty nurse, caring for a sick client or a sick family in their home, and the other the role of a community nurse, working in hospitals, shelters, or wherever the need arose.

One may argue, as noted earlier, that these men were not nurses but only provided nursing care on a temporary basis under emergency conditions. Indeed, most of these men returned to their previous occupations after a crisis had passed (Sabin, 1997). However, discounting the contribution of these men would be as foolhardy as discounting the contribution made by countless women who provided volunteer and temporary nursing care during times of war or sickness. The social mores of the times required that some men should continue to work as nurses, caring for men or the mentally ill. Sabin notes that the census records of Mississippi and Florida from the decades after the Civil War indicate that a small percentage of employed nurses were men. Nursing provided a good salary for men in tough economic times. However, the attenuation of Southern epidemics and the establishment of training schools for nursing that accepted only women led to the near extinction of male nurses in the American South by the early 20th century (Sabin, 1997).

NIGHTINGALE'S REFORMS AND THE DEMISE OF MEN IN NURSING

A number of authors have credited Florence Nightingale and her reforms with the virtual demise of men in nursing (Bartfay, 1996; Christman, 1988b; Davis & Bartfay, 2001; Evans, 2004; Mackintosh, 1997; Villeneuve, 1994). Although no one individual was more responsible for ushering in a period of female domination of nursing than Nightingale, three social changes were underway prior to Nightingale that contributed to the reduction of the number of male nurses. First, as already mentioned, there was a decline in the number of monasteries and male nursing orders combined with a relative increase in the number of convents and female nursing orders, beginning during the Renaissance. Women began to replace male clerics and laymen as nurses in many

Catholic hospitals. Second, nursing became undisciplined and of poor quality in many secular hospitals. The status of and respect for nurses, and consequently the pay, plummeted throughout northern Europe and in the former English colonies. Many nurses who were ultimately hired were social misfits, alcoholics, or ne'er-do-wells, or were prisoners or prostitutes pressed into service (Donahue, 1996; Dossey, 1999; Kalisch & Kalisch, 1986; Mackintosh, 1997). The status of nurses grew so low that it was caricatured by Charles Dickens in his Sairey Gamp and Betsy Prig characters. Although men were still required for their physical strength, in accordance with patriarchal systems that afforded men greater economic opportunities, low status–low pay positions were generally assigned to women. Consequently, the proportion of nurses who were female increased. Third, and perhaps the greatest deterrent to men in nursing prior to Nightingale, was the Industrial Revolution (Christman, 1988b; Donahue, 1996). This revolution saw the founding of numerous factories across Europe and in North America, as well as a dramatic growth in industries that extracted the natural resources needed to produce factory goods. Factories and industries required heavy physical labor and long days away from home, requirements not congruent with the female social roles of the time. Men flocked to these employment opportunities since such jobs required no formal education and paid higher wages than did farm labor or menial jobs (Christman, 1988b; Donahue, 1996).

Nightingale's ability to reform the squalid conditions in the hospitals of London arose from her success in improving the conditions of battlefield hospitals in the Crimea and India, as well as from her sociopolitical connections in England. Nightingale garnered the ire of some physicians and administrators who felt that women need only be trained as faithful maidservants and who were not used to sharing control of the patient care arena (Donahue, 1996; Dossey, 1999). The physicians and hospital administrators who allowed the poor conditions in hospitals were almost exclusively men. This fact contributed to Nightingale's view that women, by nature, were better suited for organizing, performing, and supervising the nursing care of the sick. Nightingale wrote in a letter in 1867 that

> The whole reform in nursing both at home and abroad has consisted of this: to take all power over the nursing out of the hands of men, and put it into the hands of one female trained head and make her responsible for everything. (Dossey, 1996, p. 291)

In addition, by recruiting upper-middle-class women as trained nurses, Nightingale hoped to find respectable employment for Victorian women (Bartfay, 1996; Dossey, 1999; Mackintosh, 1997), thus replacing the

"Sairey Gamp" type of nurse prevalent at the time. Nightingale established her first school for nurses at St. Thomas's Hospital in London in 1860.

The value of educated nurses in improving the care of patients was quickly recognized, and soon the demand for trained nurses blossomed. This demand prompted the expansion of Nightingale's school and created the impetus for the establishment of additional schools in England. Given Nightingale's beliefs, it is not surprising that her schools admitted only women. Initially, women were required to adhere to strict moral codes and live on the hospital premises, like women in religious orders (Kalisch & Kalisch, 1986). However, the requirements of female students and subsequent female graduates varied, and in some cases the strict regulations were loosened slightly, as schools based on the Nightingale model proliferated throughout the English-speaking world between 1870 and 1900. Many of these new schools were established and supervised by Nightingale graduates.

In England, asylums initially were able to reject the introduction of trained nurses into their sex-segregated facilities (Mackintosh, 1997). In 1879, the Medico-Psychological Association was formed by male superintendents with the goal of training and certifying male attendants. However, these attendants were ill prepared to match the respect and social acceptability of trained nurses, who generally came from a higher social class than the men. As the asylums adopted a psychiatric focus of care, attendants could not compete with female nurses who were trained in the medical model of care. Since men were barred from receiving such an education, they were relegated to the duties of orderlies (Evans, 2004; Mackintosh, 1997). Men continued to be employed as private duty nurses in England, with several associations formed in the late 19th century and early 20th century. Men were allowed to work as nurses in the British military as part of the Royal Army Medical Corps. Nearly 800 male nurses served during the Boer War (Mackintosh, 1997). However, such opportunities were not available to men in the United States. Discussion of the experiences of men in nursing in the U.S. armed forces is provided in chapter 4 of this book.

THE 20th CENTURY

The formal education of nurses moved nursing closer to the status of a profession, just as university education and/or guild membership had professionalized physicians in many European nations centuries earlier. As the number of nursing schools proliferated and as they barred men from admission, men could no longer obtain the educational resources to compete fairly for employment and recognition as nurses. In addition,

Evans (2004) notes that through much of the early 20th century, health care adopted a family model of labor division, in which predominately male occupations, such as those of physicians and pharmacists, became high-status and high-pay occupations; whereas nursing, in becoming predominately female and being associated with domestic labor, suffered low status and pay. Such gendered divisions further deterred men from nursing. In the early part of the 20th century, discriminatory registration laws in Great Britain and discriminatory military laws in the United States even further deterred men from nursing. Interestingly, educated female nurses lobbied for these discriminatory laws (Kalisch & Kalisch, 1986; Mackintosh, 1997).

In Great Britain, the Nurses Registration Act was passed in 1919 (Mackintosh, 1997). Nurse registries had begun in Great Britain as early as 1901, but this act, in effect, granted legal recognition to nurses (Kalisch & Kalisch, 2004). The registry provided the public with a way to distinguish trained nurses from those who claimed to be nurses but had not received appropriate nursing training. Only female nurses were allowed full membership on the registry. Trained male nurses were placed on a separate registry. At that time, only eight hospital schools allowed men the opportunity to receive formal training, further ensuring that their numbers in the employment pool and on the male registry would remain low. Women were often hostile toward male nurses during this time, perpetuated negative stereotypes of men in nursing, and created obstacles to their employment (Mackintosh, 1997). In response, the Society of Registered Male Nurses was formed to encourage the professional training, conduct, and tradition of men in nursing in 1937. General shortages of nurses in Britain during the years around World War II provided additional employment opportunities for men in nursing, which allowed the nursing profession and the government to witness the contributions of male nurses, particularly of those nurses serving in the British armed forces. In 1947, the sex segregation of nurse registries ended, and men were allowed education and employment equity by the 1960s. The Society of Registered Male Nurses was disbanded in 1969 following nursing reforms that improved opportunities for men; however, Mackintosh (1997) notes that negative attitudes toward men persisted, continuing to create challenges for men into the 1990s:

> the inherent beliefs in the naturalism of nursing as a woman's occupation still remained, producing two contradictory assumptions about male nurses: a) that the introduction of male nurses was an attempt in some way to violate the respectability of the occupation; and b) that because men were not naturally capable of performing caring nursing activities, male nurses could therefore not be "real" men. (p. 235)

Registration barriers for men were also present in Canada. Although registration laws varied among the provinces, it was not until 1969 that Quebec allowed men to register as nurses (Evans, 2004).

In the United States, it was the military and its restrictions that drove many men away from nursing. During the Spanish-American War, the military experienced a severe shortage of nurses to care for the sick, and employed many male and female nurses on contract. Upon the conclusion of the war, Surgeon General Sternberg was vehemently opposed to maintaining female nurses in military facilities, as he felt that corpsmen would not be able to focus on their duties if they had to work side by side with female nurses (Kalisch & Kalisch, 1986). However, influential female nurses, as well as surgeons impressed by the value of educated (and female) nurses for the sick, petitioned Congress, the War Department, and others to create the Army Nurse Corps in 1901. The corps barred men from enlistment. The Navy followed suit in 1908 with its establishment of the Navy Nurse Corps.

During World War II, the military again experienced a shortage of nurses, and recruitment calls went out to enlist female nurses. However, the military was unable to increase the number of enlisted nurses to the desired levels and was considering extending the draft to female nurses (Christman, 1988a). At the beginning of the war, the American Nurses Association, the Alumni Association of the Pennsylvania Hospital School of Nursing for Men, and individuals such as Edith Smith of the Federal Security Agency's Subcommittee on Nursing lobbied for the opportunity for men to serve as nurses in the military (Craig, 1940; Kalisch & Kalisch, 1986, 2004). An annoyed surgeon general was called before congressional committees several times, yet he stood fast to the custom of barring men from the Nurse Corps (Christman, 1988a).

Christman (1988a) notes that many male nurses wanted to work as nurses, particularly on the battlefield where female nurses were not allowed. Male nurses who enlisted or were drafted were not able to function as corpsmen "because to do so they had to go to corps school, but they were too qualified to enter that training, so they were assigned duties outside of health care" (p. 46). Christman notes that approximately 1,200 male nurses had been drafted, though none were working as nurses. One of those nurses, Jacob Rose, notes that instead of nursing, he was assigned a number of nonessential tasks, including policing empty acreage in Texas, filling roadside potholes in India, and clearing land for a baseball field (Rose, 1947). After the Battle of the Bulge, the surgeon general dropped his bill for the drafting of female nurses, and the urgency of allowing men to serve as nurses seemed to decrease as well (Christman, 1988a). It would not be until 1955, when President Eisenhower signed HR 2559, a bill introduced by Representative Frances Bolton (R-OH), that men were authorized to be commissioned as nurses in the Army and Navy Nurse Corps (Craig, 1956). That same year, Edward L. T. Lyon, a nurse anesthetist from New York, became the first man to be commissioned as a nurse in the U.S. military (*Proud to serve: The evolution of male Army Nurse Corps officers*, n.d.).

As in Great Britain, nurse registries began to appear in the United States at the dawn of the 20th century. At that time, nurses became concerned that physicians and other entrepreneurs were offering "training programs" for nurses that claimed to prepare nurses in as little as 10 weeks or through mail-order home study programs. In order to distinguish trained nurses from untrained or ill-trained nurses, registries in each of the states began to appear. Although North Carolina was the first state to create a nurse registry in 1903, it was New York's registry, adopted a few years later, that had a significant impact on future registries and curricula in nurse training programs (Kalisch & Kalisch, 2004). In New York, registration could only be achieved by graduating from a nurse training program approved by the Board of Regents of the state university. New York soon required approved programs to provide obstetrical education, a clinical topic not addressed by many schools. In order for their graduates to meet New York registration requirements, many nursing schools revised their curricula. This impacted men, in that many nursing schools barred men from obstetrical coursework or clinical experiences (Christman, 1988a), putting men at a disadvantage in passing the examinations required for course completion and/or registration.

Another factor that deterred men from nursing in the years prior to World War II was the lack of any draft deferment offered to men in nursing (Craig, 1956; Kalisch & Kalisch, 2004). Therefore, schools that accepted men as students were reluctant to do so since they could be drafted into the military at any time. Kalisch and Kalisch note that it had been recommended that the U.S. Public Health Service's Venereal Disease Department should employ 10 male nurses to assist in government investigations in the Washington, DC, area. However, when three qualified men were hired, all three were drafted. It was not until 1951 that male nursing students could receive deferments from the draft as did male students enrolled in medical or scientific programs (Craig, 1956).

Male nurses were barred from professional organizations in the early 20th century. The American Nurses Association (ANA) was founded in 1897 as the Nurses' Associated Alumnae of the United States and Canada, but the U.S. nurses separated from their Canadian colleagues and renamed themselves the ANA in 1911 (American Nurses Association, 1996; Donahue, 1996). African American nurses were eligible for membership early on, though many eventually were prevented from joining since some state associations refused them membership until

1964 (Carnegie, 1995). However, men were not allowed membership until 1930 (R. Barry, ANA Librarian, personal communication, June 21, 2005). After that time, the official position of the ANA was one of strong support of men in nursing. In 1940, the ANA formed the Men Nurses Section, and it was a strong advocate for the use of male nurses and the commissioning of male nurses in the armed forces (Craig, 1956; Kalisch & Kalisch, 2004; "Nursing in a Democracy," 1940). In a position paper from the Men Nurses Section, approved by the ANA Board of Directors in 1941, it was noted that "Men patients would receive much better care if attended by a graduate registered man nurse than by an orderly" (Kalisch & Kalisch, 2004, p. 375).

Nursing education opportunities were limited for men up to the mid-century. In 1937, some 28,000 nurses graduated from American nursing programs (Kalisch & Kalisch, 2004). However, in the academic year of 1939–1940, only 212 men were students at four accredited schools of nursing for men and 710 men at the 70 nursing schools that admitted men along with women (Craig, 1940). Despite these low numbers at the onset of World War II, Craig (1940) recounted the opportunities that awaited well-qualified young men. He noted that due to the increased need for nurses to have scientific knowledge and skills and the fact that tasks unrelated to nursing were now delegated to aides, the work of the nurse was now "more interesting and satisfying...[and] has required schools to select more capable students" (p. 666). As such, Craig recommended that

> Advisors ... carefully consider the personality, character, and ability of the prospective student. He needs to be versatile in his interests and to possess a considerable degree of leadership. There should be evidence of adequate social growth and adjustment for his age. Nursing is not a profession for a poorly adjusted or inadequate person to undertake. The young man who is well liked and respected by his fellows and by older men is the most likely to succeed. (pp. 666–667)

The opportunities awaiting men of such caliber, according to Craig, were private duty nursing, institutional nursing, industrial nursing, and special fields.

Craig (1940) made a strong pitch to encourage men to engage in private duty nursing. This came at a time when private duty nursing, once the largest specialty, was in decline due to the expansion of hospitals and in-patient care services (Kalisch & Kalisch, 2004). Craig noted that men engaged in private duty nursing often cared for clients with mental health or genito-urinary problems, and commanded higher salaries in many markets than women engaged in private duty nursing. (It is not clear whether men made higher wages due to labor inequities or whether men tended to care for clients with more challenging behavioral problems.) Craig recommended that men get themselves listed on the local state professional nursing registry in order to obtain "definite status in the local nursing field" (p. 668).

In terms of institutional nursing, Craig (1940) described the need for educated male nurses in psychiatric hospitals, noting that the care of male patients was of inferior quality when provided by male orderlies. He noted that this need was also present in general hospitals, particularly in genito-urinary units. He likened the skill level of many orderlies to that of Dickens's "Sairey Gamp." Craig noted that

> Similar care for women patients by untrained women would not be tolerated. This is where the well-trained man nurse fits into the picture. He not only renders adequate nursing care to the patient, but he is qualified to teach the orderly how to do his work in a way that assures the patient's comfort and safety. (p. 668)

Craig noted that the inequity in the care that male patients received amounted to a men's health crisis. Initially doubtful of the benefits of hiring male nurses in hospitals, administrators, such as the director of nursing of the Pennsylvania Hospital in Philadelphia, were persuaded when an improved quality of care was demonstrated after male nurses were hired. Craig also stated that working with orderlies would place male nurses in supervisory roles, which many men would find appealing.

As renewed industrialization grew in the nation at the conclusion of the Great Depression, Craig (1940) reported that 6.5% of male nursing graduates in 1939 found employment in industrial (now known as occupational health) nursing. He noted that due to the increased importance employers placed on employee health and accident reduction, industrial nursing provided excellent opportunities for steady employment. Craig recommended that men considering such employment should have an ability to work well with others, have a knowledge of how to respond to emergencies and render first aid, and have skills in typing and stenography. In terms of special fields, Craig stated that despite the opportunities mentioned, these fields were limited for men. Here, Craig advocated for the removal of curriculum barriers that prevented men from entering specialized nursing areas, such as pediatrics. Craig also advocated for the inclusion of men in military nursing and supported the efforts underway at the time to convince the government to fill vacant slots with men, particularly in the psychiatric services.

As mentioned earlier, it was not until the mid-1950s that men were allowed to serve as nurses in the military. However, decades of discrimination against men in the admission policies of nursing schools, of unequal quality of nursing curricula provided to male students, and of limited employment opportunities for male graduates took their toll, so that by 1960, only 1% of all registered nurses were male (Christman, 1988b). It is likely that this was the lowest percentage of nurses who were male since before the times of the Crusades.

In 1939, there were four all-male schools of nursing. The last of these to close was the Alexian Brothers School of Nursing for Men in Chicago in 1969 (see chapter 2). It is important to note that the school did not close due to the removal of challenges for men entering nursing school; rather, it closed along with many other diploma programs as nursing education moved to the university setting. Statistics on the number of schools that allowed men admission by decade are not available in the United States; however, Evans (2004) cites Hunter, who notes that in 1961, only 25 out of 170 schools of nursing accepted men in Canada. An important breakthrough in easing the restrictions placed on men entering nursing school came with the U.S. Supreme Court decision on July 1, 1982 in the case of Mississippi University for Women v. Hogan (Legal Information Institute, 2005), in which Justice Sandra Day O'Connor provided her first opinion for the majority as a new court justice.

In this case, Joe Hogan, an associate's-degree nurse, applied for admission to earn his bachelor's degree in nursing at Mississippi University for Women (MUW) in Columbus, MS. MUW was an all-female, publicly funded university, the only such university in Mississippi at that time. Although other Southern schools offered associate's-to-bachelor's degree programs, none were available in the local area other than MUW. Mr. Hogan was denied admission based solely on his sex and sued for violation of the Equal Protection Clause of the 14th Amendment of the U.S. Constitution. The State argued that it had a tradition and a legitimate interest in providing educational opportunities for women in sex-segregated programs. Interestingly, MUW offered Mr. Hogan the opportunity to audit the nursing courses but would not grant credit for the courses. In 1981, a time prior to Internet and media-based distance education, it is unclear how Mr. Hogan would have been able to audit the courses without being physically present in the classroom and labs. Such a presence would contradict the State's contention that an all-female environment was beneficial and important to female students.

The district court found in favor of the State, and Mr. Hogan appealed (Legal Information Institute, 2005). At the appeal, the State argued that the current policy of discrimination was a legitimate practice to counter the historical discrimination of women. The court of appeals reversed the district court's decision. This reversal was ultimately upheld by the Supreme Court. In her opinion, Justice O'Connor states that

> The State's primary justification for maintaining the single-sex admissions policy of MUW's School of Nursing is that it compensates for discrimination against women, and therefore constitutes educational affirmative action. As applied to the School of Nursing, we find the State's argument unpersuasive. (Legal Information Institute, 2005, para. 13)

In contrasting this case to precedents in which violations of the Equal Protection Clause constituted appropriate and legal actions toward affirmative action, Justice O'Connor argued that

> In sharp contrast, Mississippi has made no showing that women lacked opportunities to obtain training in the field of nursing or to attain positions of leadership in that field when the MUW School of Nursing opened its door, or that women currently are deprived of such opportunities. In fact, in 1970, the year before the School of Nursing's first class enrolled, women earned 94% of the nursing baccalaureate degrees conferred in Mississippi and 98.6% of the degrees earned nationwide. That year was not an aberration; one decade earlier, women had earned all the nursing degrees conferred in Mississippi.... Rather than compensate for discriminatory barriers faced by women, MUW's policy of excluding males from admission to the School of Nursing tends to perpetuate the stereotyped view of nursing as an exclusively woman's job. By assuring that Mississippi allots more openings in its state-supported nursing schools to women than it does to men, MUW's admissions policy lends credibility to the old view that women, not men, should become nurses, and makes the assumption that nursing is a field for women a self-fulfilling prophecy. (para. 17–18)

After this time, publicly funded schools of nursing could not indiscriminately bar men from admission. Most schools began to accept men without fanfare; however, up to the present day, many nursing schools do not routinely encourage and/or recruit men to apply or do not work with high-school guidance counselors to steer young men into considering nursing as a career (Barkley & Kohler, 1992; Kelly, Shoemaker, & Steele, 1996; O'Lynn, 2004). This topic is discussed further in chapters 13 and 14.

Despite the relatively low numbers of men entering nursing in the second half of the 20th century, men have made important contributions to the knowledge base of the profession. Pheifer and Davis (1987) noted the sex of the authors of articles published from 1955 to 1985 in three nursing journals: *Nursing Outlook,* the *American Journal of Nursing,* and *Nursing Research.* Pheifer and Davis identified 194 articles written by men. The majority of these articles published between 1955 and 1964 were submitted by administrators. Pheifer and Davis associate this finding with the Health Amendment Act of 1956, which provided federal funding for graduate nursing education in administration. Administrative positions offered leadership opportunities and higher salaries, which may have been attractive to many men. However, the topic of the majority of the articles between 1955 and 1964 was not administrative/organizational issues but direct nursing care. The employment roles of many male nurse authors shifted away from those of administrators to those of educators and clinicians over the next two decades. Pheifer and Davis associate this finding with the Nurse Training Act of 1964, which assisted graduate nursing education in education, and to the increasing numbers of men entering nursing practice. Direct nursing care remained the most common topic of the articles published between 1975 and 1984. It is not clear how these findings compare to the topics chosen by female nurse authors of the time.

Not all nurse scholars have welcomed the contributions men have made to the knowledge base of nursing. Ryan and Porter (1993) note that between 1990 and 1992, men comprised 42% of the authors for three British journals (*Nurse Education Today,* the *British Journal of Nursing,* and *Senior Nurse*) yet comprised only 9% of the registered nurse population. In the American journal, *Nursing Research,* men comprised 6% of the authors, a percentage more consistent with the percentage of men in the American registered nurse population. Ryan and Porter caution the profession that American male nurses might strive to "enjoy a disproportionate share of the access to the nursing literature" as they have done in Great Britain (p. 265). The authors imply a bias on the part of journal editors, favoring submissions by male authors. This bias is problematic, according to Ryan and Porter, since such action oppresses the feminine language and thus the feminine reality of nursing. Unfortunately, Ryan and Porter provide no evidence that bias occurs (for example, that submissions by men are disproportionately approved for publication compared with submissions by women); nor do they offer any explanation as to why men might possibly submit manuscripts at higher rates than do women.

The article by Ryan and Porter (1993) is an exemplar of how the discussion in the nursing literature of men in nursing changed after the rise of feminism. Prior to the 1970s, most articles and comments that were negative toward men adhered to beliefs that men were ill suited for nursing due to social mores, a perceived lack of caring skill, or the belief that men who pursued nursing were of questionable character.

Beginning in the 1960s, the larger feminist critique of Western society, science, and academia crept into the nursing literature. Although this critique has been useful in examining issues relevant to nursing, when directed toward the topic of men in nursing, this critique has provided a general perspective that rectification of the gender imbalance in nursing will only serve as a conduit for the introduction of patriarchal and hegemonic systems and male privilege into the profession. In order to prevent this, some feminist authors have paradoxically advocated discrimination and sexism in order to maintain the gendered status quo. Generally, men have found this position to be rather hypocritical, particularly since traditionally male-dominated health professions, such as medicine and pharmacy, have become much more gender balanced as a result of feminist advocacy and affirmative action initiatives. Some men, such as Luther Christman, have even stated that the improved gender balance of these professions was facilitated by the inherently democratic values held by men (Avery, 2001). However, criticisms from men have often been dismissed by feminist nurse authors as invalid, since men comprise an oppressing group. For example, in response to criticism of their article from Gregory Johnson and other men, Ryan and Porter argue that

> Johnson's linkage of men with oppressed minority groups demonstrates his lack of awareness of the centrality of power and inequality to minority issues. There is a need to distinguish between oppressed minorities and others. To take an historical example, in ancient Rome, slaves were in the majority and patricians in the minority. Would Johnson attack condemnation of slavery as hateful patrician-bashing? (Ryan & Porter, 1994, p. 245)

Although the appropriateness of the analogy selected by Ryan and Porter could lead to an interesting discourse, the larger issue in terms of men in nursing in the literature following the rise of feminism is the interplay between the still-present patriarchal hegemony in the larger society and the still-present matriarchal hegemony within the confines of the nursing profession. Feminist nurse scholars who focus only on the larger societal perspective fail to recognize, or possibly may condone, destructive sexism within nursing. Male critics who focus only on their experiences of discrimination or perceptions of hypocrisy within nursing fail to recognize the possibility of the inequities that they, as men, may bring to nursing. At the beginning of the 21st century, a reasoned and holistic perspective on this interplay has been lacking in the nursing literature.

LUTHER CHRISTMAN: 20TH-CENTURY NURSE LEADER, ADVOCATE, AND VISIONARY

Perhaps no other nurse in the 20th century has done more to bring visibility to the issues men have in nursing and to propose reforms that would benefit the profession as a whole than Luther Christman, RN, PhD, FAAN (Houser & Player, 2004; Sullivan, 2002). Christman was born in 1915 in a small Pennsylvania town and experienced much hard work and hardship as a child. As a teenager, he met the love of his life, Dorothy Black, who was planning to become a nurse. Upon the recommendation and assistance of his minister, Christman enrolled in the Pennsylvania Hospital School of Nursing for Men, while Dorothy enrolled in the corresponding all-female nursing school.

Throughout his career, Christman has gained notoriety for challenging the illogical nature of discriminatory beliefs and practices, often angering the nursing elite and powerful. Such confrontations started early for Christman in nursing school. As Christman (1988a) recounts:

> A similar [negative] reaction occurred when I requested a maternity experience. I submitted a request to the members of the faculty of the school for women asking to be assigned a maternity rotation so that I could be prepared in a manner akin to that of most nurses in the country. I was denied because of my gender. I questioned that because all of the obstetricians were men. Even policemen and taxicab drivers were being trained to handle emergency deliveries. "That's different," they said. I tried to persuade them that a male nurse would be more helpful in an emergency delivery than a policeman, but they were steadfast in their decision. They said that if I was ever seen anywhere near the delivery room, I would be dismissed immediately. (p. 45)

Sullivan (2002) notes that for much of his career, Christman realized that "the problems for men in nursing [were] similar to those of women in medicine; they [were] power-related" (p. 12). Instead of retreating to placid acceptance, Christman chose to advocate for greater equality in nursing from the very beginning of his career.

Christman graduated in 1939, married Dorothy, and began a long and illustrious career. Always an advocate for advanced education for nurses, Christman himself applied to earn his baccalaureate degree, but he was denied admission at Duquesne University due to his gender. He took a job outside of nursing, as it provided a better income to support his wife. Before Christman could explore other educational opportunities, World War II broke out, and Christman's first national struggle ensued: the military's ban on men serving as nurses. Christman joined the U.S.

Maritime Service and submitted a letter to the surgeon general requesting work as a nurse in the battle zone for the duration of the war.

> After what I considered a snide reply, I sent copies of my letter and his response to every US senator and about three-fourths of the members of Congress. The responses were interesting. Both Democrats and Republicans agreed that men should be commissioned.... The *Saturday Evening* Post wrote an editorial questioning the policy of not using male nurses. A column questioning that policy also appeared in the *Christian Science Monitor*. The *St. Petersburg Times* likewise ran an article that raised questions about the services' refusal to use male nurses. When the Pinnella County District Nurses Association endorsed my position, a nurse from the Army Nurse Corps subsequently appeared at one of their meetings to chide them about that move. Her position was that if men were commissioned, all the senior women nurse officers would immediately be demoted and replaced by men. (p. 46)

Although his efforts to reverse the military's discriminatory position were ultimately unsuccessful, Christman's voice contributed greatly to the debate that ensued after the war ended (Christman, 1988a; Houser & Player, 2004).

After the war, Christman again pursued his baccalaureate degree in nursing. He returned to the University of Pennsylvania, but he was told that he would receive an "F" in all of his nursing courses because he was a man and that the university would never graduate a man with a nursing degree (Christman, 1988a). He was eventually admitted to Temple University, earning his bachelor's degree in 1947. Over the next decade, Christman took positions at the Cooper Hospital School of Nursing in New Jersey and Yankton State Hospital in South Dakota. During this time, he introduced a number of reforms that increased nurses' salaries and addressed the nursing shortage by hiring corpsmen and auxiliary nursing personnel to assist with nonprofessional tasks. In South Dakota, he took bold steps, initially at great risk to himself, to provide employment opportunities to local Native American residents who were subject to great discrimination themselves (Houser & Player, 2004; Sullivan, 2002). As the 1960s approached, Christman again pursued advanced education, and he earned his master's degree in clinical psychology and his doctoral degree in anthropology and sociology from Michigan State University. While in graduate school, Christman served as the president of the Michigan Nurses' Association (MNA) and continued to fight to improve the conditions for nurses. At that time, there was a nursing shortage, and many nurses had deactivated their licenses to pursue other, better-paying employment opportunities. Christman (1988a) recounts that

One of my first acts as president of the MNA was to convene a representative group from both the MNA and the Michigan Hospital Association to examine the economic status of nurses. The meeting was long and the groups were at odds. During a break in the meeting, I went into the men's room. In that confine, an animated conversation was underway. I listened for a while, then said, "If salaries are not increased by 10%, I am calling a press conference to accuse the hospital administrators of this state of being responsible for the nurse shortage. There is little or no difference in staff salaries from hospital to hospital. I am going to accuse you folks of restraint of trade." (p. 49)

Such statements angered the administrators, but they acquiesced when Christman offered to measure the success of pay increases by the increases in the number of nurses reactivating their licenses and rejoining the nursing workforce. Within a couple of years, the number of active licensed nurses in Michigan rose from 14,000 to 21,000.

While in Michigan, Christman developed his Laws of Behavior, which he states helped him understand the seemingly irrational actions of nurse leaders and helped him roll with the punches during his career. The laws state that

1. We all want the world to be in our own image.
2. People cannot use knowledge they do not have.
3. In every instance, given the choice between rationality and irrationality, people opt for irrationality and are rational only when forced to be.
4. Most people under most circumstances will generally do what is right if they know what is right and if the temptation to err is not too great. (pp. 49–50)

At the 1964 annual convention of the American Nurses Association, Christman proposed the formation of an academy of nursing. This proposal was far ahead of its time, but Christman understood the importance such a body could have in shaping health policy and the profession. The Academy of Nursing was eventually formed in 1973; it named Christman as a "Living Legend" in 1995 (American Academy of Nursing, 2005).

After receiving his doctorate, Christman was offered and accepted the position of dean of nursing at Vanderbilt University and director of nursing at Vanderbilt Hospital in 1967. This was the first time that a man was appointed dean of a university-based school of nursing. While at Vanderbilt, Christman was the first dean to employ African American women faculty members there (American Nurses Association, 2005). Five years later, Christman was recruited to launch the Rush University School of Nursing and serve as its dean. While serving in these two positions,

Christman accomplished a great deal to advance the nursing profession, including the following:

1. He adopted and refined the faculty-practice model, in which faculty spent the majority of their time working as expert clinicians, in a fashion similar to that of the faculty of most medical schools.
2. He created the unification model of nursing education, which incorporated the model of faculty practice and in which graduate nursing students studied side by side with medical students, so that each might learn from and gain respect for each other's disciplines.
3. He planted the seeds for the development of a clinical master's degree that would prepare nurses for advanced practice.
4. He was responsible for the development of the primary nurse model of care.
5. He obtained numerous grants to implement innovative models of nursing education and support nursing research.
6. He developed the combined DNSc/PhD doctoral program in order to develop strong nurse scholars.
7. He founded a community nursing service that provided continuity of care to medical center clients. (Christman, 1988a; Houser & Player, 2004; Sullivan, 2002)

These accomplishments were revolutionary for the time, and not all of Christman's proposals were well received by the nursing elite. For example, Christman proposed a clinical master's degree in psychiatry to prepare advanced nurse clinicians. He consulted with Dr. Ewald Busse, a psychiatrist from Duke University, to develop a program at Duke that would adopt the tenets of the unification model of interdisciplinary education and practice. However, when the National League for Nursing was informed of this proposal, it threatened to rescind Duke University's accreditation if the proposal was implemented. Christman and his team appealed to the American Nurses Association for support but received none. The physicians believed strongly in the benefits of a highly educated mid-level practitioner. Since nursing was not willing to move in that direction at that time, the physicians developed a physician's assistant program instead (Houser & Player, 2004). One can only imagine how the decades-long tension between nurse practitioners, physicians, and physicians' assistants might have been affected had nursing adopted Christman's integrated and collaborative proposal instead of waiting years to implement widespread clinical graduate nursing education.

Eventually, many of Christman's ideas were adopted by nursing, but only years after Christman had proposed them.

One of Christman's legacies is the formation of the American Assembly for Men in Nursing in 1974. Three years earlier, Christman had been invited to help in the organization of a group for Michigan male nurses. This group eventually foundered, but Christman reconvened the group in Chicago in 1974 as the National Male Nurses Association, which was renamed the American Assembly for Men in Nursing (AAMN) in 1980. At its inception, the purpose of the group was to foster the recruitment of more men into nursing. Christman remains the chairman of the board of AAMN to this day. (The development and growth of the AAMN is the topic of chapter 3.) Christman retired in 1987, yet he has remained active in professional nursing and science organizations. In 2004, Christman was the first (and to this date, the only) man to be inducted into the American Nurses Association Hall of Fame (American Nurses Association, 2005).

CONCLUSION

Genealogy is an enjoyable hobby and, for some, a passionate undertaking. This activity seems to be growing if one takes note of the increasing number of books, Web sites, and conferences devoted to the subject. For those pursing personal genealogical knowledge, motivation comes not only from a curiosity about one's family history but also from a deep-seated need to understand one's historical identity and place in the world. And so it is for men who are nurses. Men have a deep-seated need to understand their historical identities as nurses. Men also have a deep-seated need to be proud of their historical contributions. Such an understanding and such a pride have been difficult to develop, since many nurse educators and historians have provided only a cursory summary, if any at all, of our rich history.

Anecdotally, male nursing students have gazed at photographs of Florence Nightingale, Clara Barton, and Lillian Wald and asked, "How do these women relate to me?" Although the students understand the important accomplishments of these women, some male students find it difficult to transfer inspiration from these women into the gendered realities of their lives and of today's nurses. In addition, male students find some nameless crusader an inadequate role model as they develop their own professional identities. In far too few pages, this chapter has attempted to provide a helpful summary of the rich history of men in nursing spanning some 2,000 years. But in these pages, identifiable historical role models for men, such as Brother Gerard, Camillus de Lellis, and Luther Christman, as well as the countless lay and religious brethren who tended to the sick and the poor, are offered. In understanding these historical figures, men can look at today's male role models and nursing leaders, some of whom have contributed chapters to this book, with a greater sense of appreciation and honor.

Historically, men have worn multiple hats: soldier and nurse, cleric and nurse, author/poet and volunteer nurse. Similarly, women have worn multiple hats: suffragette and nurse, nun and nurse, housewife and volunteer nurse. Admirable individuals from all walks of life have worked as nurses worthy of role-model status over the centuries. Today, nurses of either gender should be inspired by and respectful of any person from the past who, through compassion and caring, has mopped the sweaty brow of a suffering human being.

REFERENCES

Alexian Brothers. (2005). *Early history of the Alexian Brothers.* Retrieved October 20, 2005, from http://www.alexianbrothers.org/english/history/timeline.html

American Academy of Nursing. (2005). *Living legends.* Retrieved November 6, 2005, from http://www.aannet.org/fellowship/II/history.asp

American Nurses Association. (1996). *In the beginning.* Retrieved November 7, 2005, from http://nursingworld.org/centenn/centbegn.htm

American Nurses Association. (2005). *ANA Hall of Fame.* Retrieved November 10, 2005, from http://nursingworld.org/hof/alphalst.htm

AmeriCares. (2003). *AmeriCares assists needy in El Salvador, Guatemala.* Retrieved October 7, 2005, from http://www.americares.org/newsroom/?id = 21

Avery, C. T. P. (2001). A conversation with Luther: The opinions and predictions of Dr. Luther Christman [Videotape].

Bainbridge, D. (2001). Disappointed in article on men in nursing. *Canadian Nurse, 97*(7), 7–8.

Barkley, T. W., & Kohler, P. A. (1992). Is nursing's image a deterrent to recruiting men into the profession? Male high school students respond. *Nursing Forum, 27*(2), 9–13.

Bartfay, W. J. (1996). A "masculinist" historical perspective of nursing. *Canadian Nurse, 92*(2), 17–18.

Bullough, V. L. (1994). Men in nursing. *Journal of Professional Nursing, 10*(5), 267.

Bullough, V. L., & Bullough, B. (1993). Medieval nursing. *Nursing History Review, 1,* 89–104.

Carnegie, M. E. (1995). *The path we tread: Blacks in nursing worldwide 1854–1994.* New York: NLN Press.

Catholic Community Forum. (2002). *Patron saint index.* Retrieved June 21, 2002, from http://www.catholic-forum.com/saints/pst00524.htm

Christman, L. (1988a). Luther Christman. In T. M. Schoor & A. Zimmerman (Eds.), *Making choices, taking chances: Nurse leaders tell their stories* (pp. 43–52). St. Louis, MO: The C. V. Mosby Company.

Christman, L. (1988b). Men in nursing. *Annual Review of Nursing Research, 6,* 193–205.

Craig, L. N. (1940). Opportunities for men nurses. *American Journal of Nursing, 40*(6), 666–670.

Craig, L. N. (1956). Another goal achieved. *Nursing Outlook, 4*(3), 175–176.

Davis, M. T., & Bartfay, W. J. (2001). Men in nursing: An untapped resource. *Canadian Nurse, 97*(5), 14–18.

Donahue, M. P. (1996). *Nursing: The finest art: An illustrated history* (2nd ed.). St. Louis, MO: Mosby.

Dossey, B. M. (1999). *Florence Nightingale: Mystic, visionary, healer.* Springhouse, PA: Springhouse Corporation.

Evans, J. (2004). Men nurses: A historical and feminist perspective. *Journal of Advanced Nursing, 47*(3), 321–328.

Gomez, A. (1994). Men in nursing: An historical perspective. *Nurse Educator, 19*(5), 13–14.

Goodier, A. (1959). *Saints for sinners.* Retrieved October 29, 2005, from http://www.ewtn.com/library/MARY/STCAML.htm

Hospitaller Brothers of St. John of God. (2005). *Hospitaller Brothers of St. John of God* [Homepage]. Retrieved October 29, 2005, from http://www.stjohnofgod.org

Houser, B. P., & Player, K. N. (2004). *Pivotal moments in nursing: Leaders who changed the path of a profession.* Indianapolis, IN: Sigma Theta Tau International.

Kalisch, P. A., & Kalisch, B. J. (1986). *The advance of American nursing* (2nd ed.). Boston: Little, Brown & Company.

Kalisch, P. A., & Kalisch, B. J. (2004). *American nursing: A history* (4th ed.). Philadelphia: Lippincott Williams & Wilkins.

Kelly, N. R., Shoemaker, M., & Steele, T. (1996). The experience of being a male student nurse. *Journal of Nursing Education, 35*(4), 170–174.

Knight, K. (2005a, October 6, 2005). *Catholic Encyclopedia: Brothers Hospitallers of St. John of God.* Retrieved October 29, 2005, from http://www.newadvent.org/cathen/02802b.htm

Knight, K. (2005b, October 6, 2005). *Catholic Encyclopedia: Order of St. Lazarus of Jerusalem.* Retrieved October 29, 2005, from http://www.newadvent.org/cathen/09096b.htm

Knight, K. (2005c, October 6, 2005). *Catholic Encyclopedia: Orders of Saint Anthony.* Retrieved October 20, 2005, from http://www.newadvent.org/cathen/01555a.htm

Knight, K. (2005d, October 6, 2005). *Catholic Encyclopedia: Orders of the Holy Spirit.* Retrieved October 29, 2005, from http://www.newadvent.org/cathen/07415a.htm

Knight, K. (2005e, October 6, 2005). *Catholic Encyclopedia: St. Basil the Great.* Retrieved October 20, 2005, from http://www.newadvent.org/cathen/02330b.htm

Knight, K. (2005f, October 6, 2005). *Catholic Encyclopedia: St. John of God.* Retrieved October 29, 2005, from http://www.newadvent.org/cathen/08472c.htm

Lascaratos, J., Kalantzis, G., & Poulakou-Rebelakou, E. (2004). Nursing homes for the old ("Gerocomeia") in Byzantium (324–1453 AD). *Gerontology, 50,* 113–117.

Legal Information Institute. (2005). *458 US 718: Mississippi University for Women v. Hogan.* Retrieved July 9, 2005, from http://straylight.law.cornell.edu/supct/html/historics/USSC_CR_0458_0718_ZO.html

Mackintosh, C. (1997). A historical study of men in nursing. *Journal of Advanced Nursing, 26*(2), 232–236.

Mellish, J. M. (1990). *A basic history of nursing* (2nd ed.). Durban, South Africa: Butterworth's.

Murthy, K. R. S. (1994). *Vagbhata's Astangahrdayam: Text, English translation, notes, appendix and indices: Volume I: Sutrasthana and sarira sthana.* Varanasi, India: Krishnadas Academy.

Nursing in a democracy. (1940). *American Journal of Nursing, 40*(6), 671–672.

Nutting, M. A., & Dock, L. L. (1935). *A history of nursing.* New York: G. P. Putnam's Sons.

O'Lynn, C. E. (2004). Gender-based barriers for male students in nursing education programs: Prevalence and perceived importance. *Journal of Nursing Education, 43*(5), 229–236.

Opsahl, E. (1996). *Chronological table of events: Teutonic Knights.* Retrieved October 24, 2005, from http://www.the-orb.net/encyclop/religion/monastic/opsahl2.html

Pheifer, W. G., & Davis, L. L. (1987). Men in nursing: Their contributions to the mainstream nursing literature, 1955–1985. *Journal of Nursing History, 3*(1), 5–16.

Pokorny, M. E. (1992). An historical perspective of confederate nursing during the Civil War, 1861–1865. *Nursing Research, 41*(1), 29.

Proud to serve: The evolution of male Army Nurse Corps officers. (n.d.). Retrieved October 21, 2005, from http://history.amedd.army.mil/ANCWebsite/articles/malenurses.htm

Rose, J. (1947). Men nurses in military service. *American Journal of Nursing, 47*(3), 146.

Ryan, S., & Porter, S. (1993). Men in nursing: A cautionary comparative critique. *Nursing Outlook, 41*(6), 262–267.

Ryan, S., & Porter, S. (1994). Men in nursing: Reply to letter to the editor. *Nursing Outlook, 42*(5), 244–247.

Sabin, L. E. (1997). Unheralded nurses. Male care givers in the nineteenth-century south. *Nursing History Review, 5,* 131–148.

Sapountzi-Krepia, D. (2004, April–June). European nursing history: Nursing care provision and nursing training in Greece and ancient times until the creation of the modern Greek state [Electronic version]. *ICUs and Nursing Web Journal, 18,* 1–4.

Sire, H. J. A. (1994). *The Knights of Malta.* New Haven, CT: Yale University Press.

Sovereign Order of Malta. (2005). *History.* Retrieved October 7, 2005, from http://www.orderofmalta.org/storia.asp?idlingua = 5

Sterns, I. (1969). *Military Orders: The rule and statutes of the Teutonic Knights.* Retrieved October 24, 2005, from http://www.the-orb.net/encyclop/religion/monastic/tk_rule.html

Sullivan, E. (2002, Third Quarter). In a woman's world. *Reflections on Nursing Leadership,* 10–17.

Villeneuve, M. J. (1994). Recruiting and retaining men in nursing: A review of the literature. *Journal of Professional Nursing, 10*(4), 217–228.

Wilson, B. (1997, November 5). *Men in American nursing history.* Retrieved April 8, 2002, from http://www.geocities.com/Athens/Forum/6011/sld003.htm

Zinn, H. (2003). *A people's history of the United States: 1492–present.* New York: HarperCollins.

CHAPTER TWO

American Schools of Nursing for Men

Russell E. Tranbarger

INTRODUCTION

Walk down any street in America and stop people at random. Ask them to describe a *nurse* to you. Almost always the description will be of a female person possessing traits generally associated with females. Interestingly, prior to the 20th century, nursing was as often practiced by men as it was by women. For at least 1,000 years, nursing care was provided by Catholic religious orders in monasteries and convents to sick and injured people. Wilson (1997) reports that nursing care was provided during the Crusades by the Knights Templar and other groups to sick and injured crusaders. The Congregation of Alexian Brothers, a religious congregation still active today, records in its history the care and burial of victims of the bubonic plague in Europe (Alexian Brothers, 2005a). More recently, during the U.S. Civil War, more than 50% of the individuals contracted to provide nursing services to the Union forces were men (E. Halloran, personal communication, 2005). Pokorny (1992) notes that men were employed as nurses by both the Union forces and the Confederacy; but most of the literature has focused on the women who were volunteers for the Union. Pokorny also identified Walt Whitman as a nurse during the U.S. Civil War. Walt Whitman, in his collection of poetry, *Leaves of Grass* (1865/1975), includes a poem entitled "The Wound Dresser," thought to have evolved from his work as a nurse during the Civil War.

Although the first known formal school of nursing, established about 250 b.c. in India, admitted only men students (Wilson, 1997), Florence

43

Nightingale is credited with the development of modern nursing education. As her fame grew and the Nightingale model of schools of nursing (in which only female students were allowed admission) developed and spread around the world, nursing became the province of women. Thus, Nightingale is probably responsible for the feminization of modern nursing. It is reasonable to accept that in the Victorian era in which she lived, Nightingale's desire to create an acceptable role for women outside of marriage and home necessitated showing either that men were unsuitable for the role of nurse or that it would be inappropriate for men to function as nurses. It is fair to say that Nightingale proved her point and succeeded wildly!

Problems soon arose, however. As nursing training schools expanded and improved the nursing care of patients, doctors began to witness the evolution of two standards of care: one for women and another for men. The modern nursing model was predicated on Victorian culture. Thus, women demurely turned the intimate care of male patients over to less adequately trained orderlies, while providing intimate nursing care to females. Physicians in the United States soon began to complain about differences in the care provided to their patients.

Another dilemma of this era was the absence of medications, especially tranquilizers, for the treatment of the mentally ill. Patients were hospitalized in mental institutions and were segregated by sex. This resulted in the staffing of female units by trained nurses and students, while the male wards were staffed by orderlies and attendants. Some supervision of the male units was provided by nurses, but the care was delegated to the less adequately trained male employees and "trusties," those patients showing an improvement in their condition. The first efforts to address this issue of different care for different genders resulted in programs to educate orderlies in simple nursing procedures. The results left much to be desired, and physicians continued to call for improvements in the care of male patients.

By the late 19th century, a few schools of nursing for men had been opened in the United States. Table 2.1 lists some of the schools of nursing for men that have been noted in the literature. It is likely that other schools operated during the 20th century, but their history is less well known. The remainder of this chapter will provide historical and personal accounts of some of these schools.

THE MILLS TRAINING SCHOOL FOR MEN

In 1888, the Mills Training School for Men opened to train men to work in the men's wards of Bellevue Hospital, New York. Dr. Mills, a dentist and philanthropist, donated the money to build the school. The Mills Training program grew, and jealousies between the school for women

TABLE 2.1   Schools of Nursing for Men in the United States

Date opened	School	Location
1886	School for Male Nurses	Blackwell's Welfare Island, NY
1886	McLean Hospital School of Nursing for Men	Waverly, MA
1888	Mills Training School for Men	Bellevue Hospital, New York City
1888	St. Vincent Hospital School for Men	New York City
1898	Alexian Brothers Hospital School of Nursing	Chicago, IL
1914	Pennsylvania Hospital School of Nursing	Philadelphia, PA
1928	Alexian Brothers Hospital School of Nursing	St. Louis, MO
1929	St. Joseph's Hospital School of Nursing	New York City

and the training program for men also grew. In 1910 the Mills Training School was closed, possibly due to the death of a patient on the men's psychiatry ward. The school then began to train men as orderlies. The Mills Training School reopened in 1920, and in 1929 the two nursing schools for men and for women were merged under a single administration as the Bellevue Schools of Nursing (Bellevue Alumnae Association Collection, 2004).

The Mills School for Men closed during World War II and reopened once more in 1948. In 1954, the schools of nursing joined the newly formed National Student Nurses Association (NSNA), and Joseph Barry, Mills Class of 1954, was elected the first recording secretary of the NSNA (Bellevue Alumnae Association Collection, 2004). In 1957, a change in the curriculum permitted men students to study obstetric nursing, which included clinical assignments. In 1958 the schools were renamed the Bellevue and Mills Schools of Nursing. No students were admitted after 1967 and both diploma programs closed in 1969.

It should also be noted that a graduate of the Mills Training School for men, L. Bissell Sanford, was appointed to the first New York State Board of Examiners of Registered Nurses when it was established late in 1903. He was in the first group of nurses in New York to become registered nurses. He earned the title of the first man to become a registered nurse in the United States (New York State Board of Examiners of Registered Nurses, 1905).

THE ALEXIAN BROTHERS HOSPITAL SCHOOL OF NURSING

The Chicago School

The fifth school of nursing for men was opened in Chicago in 1898. The program was developed to train the members of the Congregation of Alexian Brothers, a Catholic religious group of men. As noted earlier, the congregation has a long history, and recently discovered documents in Belgium indicate its existence there in 1057 (Alexian Brothers, personal communication, 1999). The congregation came to prominence during the times of the Black Death, or plague, when the dead and dying were abandoned where they fell. The brothers served a public health need by collecting and burying the dead. Thus, their original charism was the preparation of the dead for burial, the preparation of the grave, the conducting of the burial service, and the care of the grave after the burial. They were paid by the city fathers for these services. Their coat of arms to this date includes a pair of crossed shovels signifying this aspect of their history, which continued until late in the 20th century (Alexian Brothers, 2005a) (see Figure 2.1). As the plague waned, the brothers began to care for those still alive. They discovered the need for extra work during periods of declining health prior to death, and began to care for sick men. Much of the care was provided in the sick person's home. The indigent were brought to the monastery and cared for there. The brothers began their work as the first funeral directors, and then segued into public health, home nursing, and psychiatric care (Kauffman, 1976).

The brothers came to America in the 19th century and settled in Chicago (Alexian Brothers, 2005b; Kaufman, 1976). Their first hospital burned down in the Great Chicago Fire of 1871, and they eventually settled on the north side of the city (see Figure 2.2). The brothers demanded that the care they provided, even when primarily charitable in nature, be of the highest professional caliber. Thus, they hired E. H. Hearst, a graduate of the Mills Training School for Men Class of 1898, to serve as the superintendent of nursing and to open a school of nursing to train the brothers (Alexian Brothers, 2002). The brothers fired him after the first year, and from that time on, the superintendent of nursing, later called the director of nursing, was always a member of the congregation.

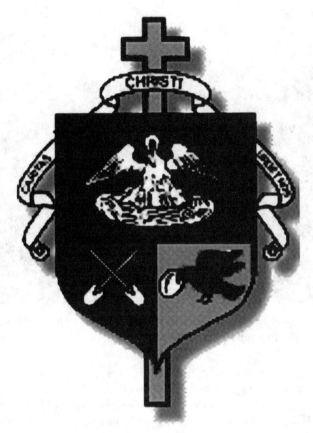

FIGURE 2.1   Coat of arms of the Alexian Brothers. © Alexian
Brothers, by permission.

During World War I, the brothers determined they needed to expand
their facilities, both at the hospital and at the school of nursing. They
appealed to the American Legion for support and assistance. The effort
failed on a vote, but the brothers garnered individual support and moved
ahead with their expansion plans. In 1925, nursing in Illinois began to
identify the need for standardization of the curriculum in all of its nursing schools. On April 1, 1925, the State of Illinois accredited the Alexian
Brothers' program and specified the number of hours to be given to each
subject. The faculty of the school was organized as a distinct unit in 1927
for the intended purpose of identifying and resolving problems with the
program of instruction. In October 1932, the State of Illinois certified the
school with certificate number 2, indicating that it was the second school

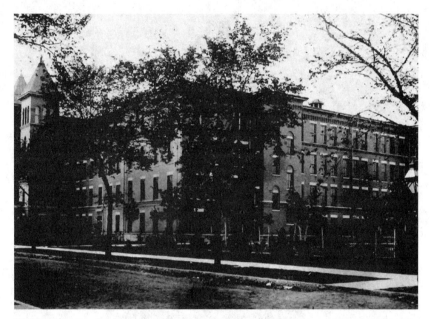

FIGURE 2.2   Alexian Brothers Hospital, Chicago, circa 1898.
© Alexian Brothers, by permission.

of nursing in Illinois to be certified. The period of the Great Depression
(1929–1940) created problems for the brothers. The numbers of patients
in the hospitals fell, as did the financial resources, but the brothers held
firm to their mission to care for the sick and poor and maintained the
services, including the school.

By 1939, the financial circumstances began to show some improvement, and the brothers made two decisions regarding the school of
nursing. First, they decided to admit the first laymen to the nursing program. The second decision was to establish an affiliation with DePaul
University. The agreement with DePaul was reached in March 1939. On
September 7, 1939, 27 students were enrolled, including the first group
of lay students.

World War II caused issues for the school. The draft board refused to
grant deferments for the students except for six months at a time. Consequently, the brothers decided to suspend admission to the school from
1942 to 1945. Conscientious objectors were assigned to the brothers
and provided staffing assistance during this period. Delegations from the
brothers and the Alumni Association made frequent trips to the Illinois
legislature in Springfield and to Washington, DC, to lobby for change in
the Army-Navy Nurses Act to permit registered male nurses to be commissioned in the Nurse Corps. They continued to be strong advocates for

this change until the federal bill sponsored by Congresswoman Frances P. Bolton (R-OH) was passed in August 1955 and signed into law.

During the 1950s, the brothers focused on strengthening the curriculum. Affiliations (clinical agreements) were established in psychiatric nursing at the Alexian Brothers Hospital in St. Louis, MO (12 weeks). A 12-week pediatric affiliation was arranged with Children's Memorial Hospital, Chicago, on March 24, 1952, for lay students. A different affiliation agreement for the student brothers was reached with St. Frances Hospital in Evanston, IL. An 8-week affiliation in tuberculosis nursing was signed with the Municipal Tuberculosis Sanitarium, Chicago, in 1951. The National League for Nursing granted temporary accreditation for the school on May 12, 1952, and granted full accreditation in 1956. The new school of nursing residence hall and classrooms were officially dedicated by His Eminence Cardinal Samuel Stritch on October 9, 1955 (see Figure 2.3). The first general reunion of all classes was also held in 1955.

Other curricular changes occurred in the 1950s. The first was the employment of an athletic director and a librarian when the school's new residence hall was occupied. A gymnasium with a stage and a swimming pool in the basement led to swimming becoming a cocurricular requirement for all students. An effort was made to reduce the heavy workload of the first-year students by initiating a concurrent teaching program and

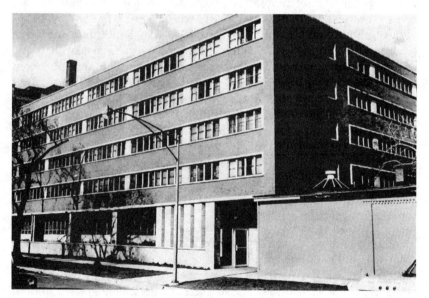

FIGURE 2.3   Alexian Brothers Hospital School of Nursing for Men, Chicago, 1956. © Alexian Brothers, by permission.

a summer session. The areas of medical, surgical, urological, dermato-logical, and venereal disease, orthopedic nursing, operating room tech-nique, and diet therapy were included in this venture (see appendix to this chapter).

The school continued to grow in size and peaked in 1962 when 13 full-time faculty members and 8 lecturers educated a class of 42 students. Beginning in the 1960s, many nursing programs were moving to the university setting. The brothers, always advocates for excellence in education, decided to close the school, in accordance with this trend, in December 1966. The final class graduated in August 1969, becoming the last cohort of students from the last remaining school of nursing for men in the United States. During the years when the schools operated in St. Louis and Chicago, 1,002 brothers and laymen graduated from the nursing programs (Alexian Brothers, 2002).

A Personal Account of Student Nurse Life in the 1950s at the Chicago School

We prospective students were required to visit the school of nursing in Chicago and experience two days of testing and interviews. Aptitude, in-telligence testing, and interviews by faculty members and upperclassmen created an applicant's database, along with transcripts and letters of rec-ommendation. Out of almost 300 prospective students, 55 students were chosen for the Class of 1959. We entered the school on Labor Day, 1956! I always thought it prophetic that Labor Day was the entrance date since labor was a large part of the educational process. The cost of the three years of nursing school, including books, laboratory fees, tuition, room and board, uniforms, laundry, and so forth amounted to $375. I received no stipends, but I did 44 hours of work per week including class.

Upon arrival, we were assigned rooms, given directions to the loca-tions of mail boxes, informed of the cafeteria hours, and told to appear for our first class at 7 p.m. After more orientation information and intro-ductions, we were notified that the entire class would produce a "talent show" three days hence for the faculty and upperclassmen. This forced us to quickly get acquainted, identify leaders in our group, and begin the quest to remain enrolled in the program. Also that day, we received class assignments and books, were measured for uniforms, and so on. The uniforms arrived in about two weeks, and we were required to wear them to all classes and official functions. We also began an introduc-tion to the clinical experience. We were assigned to nursing units for a week on each unit, then we were assigned to individual units for a month each. Upon completion of the first semester of school, those of us who remained in the program (now about 45 students) were notified that we had successfully completed our preclinical phase and were given our first "blue diamond" pin (see Figure 2.4). A ceremony was held with family and friends invited to observe the receipt of this pin and the recitation of the Nightingale Pledge.

We were granted our first vacation from school at the Christmas holiday season. Half of the class received the week of Christmas off; the other half received the week of New Year's Day off. We then received a 2-week vacation sometime during the summer and received our second blue diamond pin, signifying that we were now "junior students." Individual students began affiliations and each of us received a rotation for the remainder of our student time. We were required to document the types of patients we cared for, the number of patients, hours worked, and so forth. A blur of work, class, student activities, and mandatory

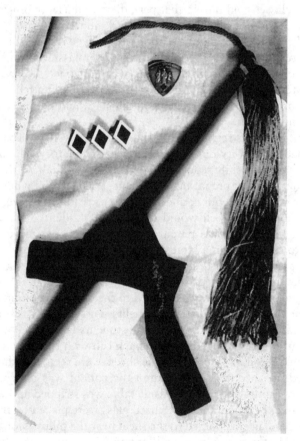

FIGURE 2.4   Alexian Brothers Hospital School of Nursing for Men blue diamond pins. © Alexian Brothers, by permission.

study hours filled the 24 hours. The rules for men students were slightly relaxed compared to those of our female cohorts in other nursing programs. We had one overnight pass each week in the first year, and these passes gradually increased until they were unlimited. However, we had to be in the school by midnight or remain outside the residence hall until 6 a.m.!

Our clinical hours in the first year were 7–10 a.m. and 3–6 p.m. daily, including most weekends. We were required to work 44 hours each week, including class hours. By the end of the first year, our classes were reduced considerably and our clinical hours increased commensurately. We were required to work at least one nightshift assignment, which lasted from 9 p.m. to 7 a.m. We received a week free of clinical work prior to and following the nightshift assignment. During the night assignment, we worked 7 nights a week for 2 weeks. In addition, we were expected to attend any classes held during that period, as well as any official student meetings that did not conflict with our work hours.

Another interesting part of school life involved respect for others. As first-year students, we were required to do upperclassmen's laundry upon request. We were also required to stand when anyone who had seniority over us entered the nursing unit. All brothers (including fellow students who were brothers), all upperclassmen, all staff, and all physicians were accorded this respect.

Patient care was regimented in those days as well. Every patient received a bed bath every day, even if he was ambulatory. The day began with the change of shift report at 6:45 a.m. Then, half of the students went through the unit preparing the patients for breakfast while the other half took temperature, pulse, and respirations readings of every patient. At about 7:30 a.m., a bell would ring and all students reported to the "floor" kitchen. Food was prepared in the main hospital kitchen and delivered to each floor in a large cart. The charge nurse would call each patient's name and food desires, while an assembly line of students assembled the tray and placed it on a delivery cart. When all the food trays had been prepared, the cart was pushed to the appropriate unit and trays were taken to the correct patient. Patients who needed assistance were fed. After all the patients had eaten, the students began the "a.m. care." Each patient received a bed bath and back rub with lotion and was then gotten out of bed if at all possible; the sheets were removed, the mattress was flipped, the bed was remade, and the patient was returned to bed unless he was ambulatory. The bedside table was stripped and washed. A fresh container of water and a sterilized glass were placed on the cleaned table. A paper bag was pinned to the sheet near the pillow along with the call button. The window ledge and footstool were washed. After all this was completed, the student proceeded to the next patient. By 10 a.m., all patient care and charting were to have been completed, and first-year students left for class. However if a student's work was not completed, the student had to remain until it was. If a student was late for class, he had to go to the director's office and explain why he had been unable to complete his assignment on time. As in the military, excuses were seldom accepted!

Student life also had moments of pleasure. Each student was required to become a proficient swimmer. Basketball, touch football, tennis, table tennis, and boxing were organized intramurally and also as "pick-up" games. Generally once a month, a dance or carnival was held, with invitations extended to female nursing students from nearby schools. Every student was also a member of the Student Nurse Association of Illinois and the National Student Nurses Association. When 30 or 40 men from the Alexian Brothers showed up at a student association meeting or function, a good time was had by all!

The school established several affiliations to provide its students with opportunities to care for women and children. An affiliation agreement with the Children's Memorial Hospital was signed on March 24, 1952, for lay students (Alexian Brothers, 2005b). At that time, many schools of nursing were affiliated there, from all over Illinois and surrounding states. In 1959, when I completed 12 weeks of pediatrics there, some of the rules still seemed archaic. For example, for the first 6 weeks of the affiliation, the student was considered a "junior" student, while for the last 6 weeks, the student was considered a "senior" student. This designation had nothing to do with actual class rank in the student's school of nursing but referred only to time spent in the affiliation. Only "senior" students were permitted to do charge duty. However, men students were declared "senior" students at the end of the second week of the experience. Men students could be assigned children of either sex under the age of 18 months or over the age of 12. However, male students could care for boy patients only when the child was between 18 months and 12 years of age.

Prior to 1958, the Illinois Board of Nursing required men students to study the theory of obstetrics but did not require clinical experience in obstetrics. When men took the licensing examination, they could elect to take the traditional five-part exam in medical, surgical, psychiatric, pediatric, and obstetric nursing, or they could substitute a written exam in urology for the obstetric portion. The rules were changed in 1958, and all students were required to have clinical experience in obstetrics and take the full examination. Cardinal Stritch, Archbishop of Chicago, had to negotiate for the obstetrics experience for the students at Alexian Brothers when all the hospitals with active delivery services refused to accept men nursing students. My affiliation was at Mercy Hospital on

the south side of Chicago, and my instructor was Sister Annette. We were
given several rules to follow:

1. We must never tell anyone we were nursing students; we were to
    say we were in medical school.
2. We had two weeks in Labor/Delivery. We were placed in the
    Doctors' Dressing Room until "crowning" and then ushered
    into the labor room and allowed to observe until delivery oc-
    curred. We were then allowed to take the new mother to post-
    partum, take the baby to the newborn nursery, clean the delivery
    room, prepare it for the next delivery, and then return to the
    Doctors' Dressing Room.
3. During the time assigned to postpartum, we were assigned to
    administer oral medications only.
4. While assigned to the clinics, we were treated as professional
    nursing students. We were encouraged to take pelvimetry mea-
    surements, listen to fetal heart tones, assist with any procedures
    performed, and so forth.
5. Throughout the 12 weeks of the experience, which was on the
    day shift, we were encouraged to work an 8-hour shift for the
    hospital, to assist in their staffing needs. We were paid well for
    these hours and I worked often. Most of my staffing there was
    during the evening hours on what would be called a step-down
    neurological unit today. Most of the patients were female, all
    were comatose, all required intimate care, all were on tube feed-
    ings, and so on. It was a marvel to me to see how differently I
    was treated in the same facility, depending on whether I was
    there as a student or as a staff member.

The St. Louis School

The brothers recognized the need to train more men as nurses, since the
administration of the congregation continued to restrict admission to the
Chicago program to their own members and to refuse admission to laymen. Consequently, they opened the school in St. Louis as a section of the
St. Louis University School of Nursing. The section was restricted to men,
and laymen were admitted to the school beginning in September 1928
under the direction of Brother Camillus Snyder. The school was considered a unit of St. Louis University. The number of applications exceeded
the number that could be admitted, and so the program prospered. After
1933, the school's status changed to that of a school affiliated with St.
Louis University, but it was effectively run by the brothers. The advent of
World War II caused the school to suspend admissions. The first postwar

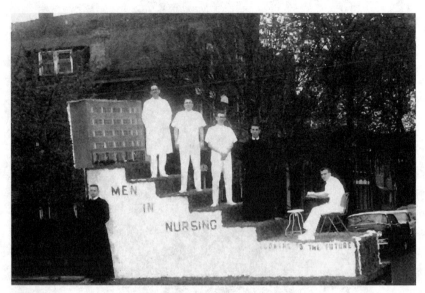

FIGURE 2.5   Alexian Brothers' float for the Nurse Day Parade,
Chicago, 1957. Photograph from Russell E. Tranbarger, by permission.

class was admitted in 1949 and consisted of 17 students. In 1951, the
St. Louis school merged with the larger program in Chicago (Alexian
Brothers, 2005c).

THE PENNSYLVANIA HOSPITAL SCHOOL OF NURSING
FOR MEN

The Pennsylvania Hospital in Philadelphia was founded in 1751 by
Benjamin Franklin and Dr. Thomas Bond. It has been recognized as
an innovator in care since its beginning (University of Pennsylvania
Health System, 2005a). A school of nursing for women only was established in 1875 and operated until 1974. It co-trained nurses from the
Women's Hospital of Philadelphia until 1882 when the independent
school of nursing was reestablished. The school established a prec-
edent when, in 1885, three female nurses were assigned to render care
to men patients on the male medical wards (University of Pennsylvania
Health System, 2005b).

The School of Nursing for Men was opened in 1914 at the Depart-
ment of Mental and Nervous Diseases, located at the hospital's West
Philadelphia campus. Leroy N. Craig was employed to lead the school.
Mr. Craig was a graduate of the Mclean Hospital School of Nursing for

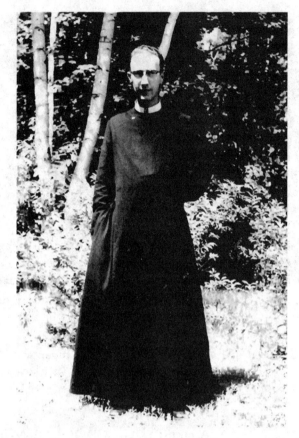

FIGURE 2.6   Brother Maurice Wilson, CFA, Director of Alexian
Brothers Hospital School of Nursing, Chicago, 1953–1969. © Alexian
Brothers, by permission.

Men in Waverly, MA. "The purpose of the school was to meet the needs of
the Philadelphia community for competent professional male nurses. The
program was designed to provide an integrated background in general
nursing upon which specialization in psychiatric and urological nursing
could be developed after completion of the course" (University of Pennsylvania Health System, 2005c, para. 3). In 1932, an affiliate program in
psychiatric nursing was created with eight other diploma programs along
with the school for men. Approximately 12,000 students were affiliated
through this effort (University of Pennsylvania Health System, 2005c).
In the 1950s, Mr. Craig worked with Congresswoman Frances P. Bolton
(R-OH) to provide for the commissioning of men registered nurses in the

military nurse corps (University of Pennsylvania Health System, 2005c). The School of Nursing for Men was dissolved in 1965, having graduated 551 men over its 51-year history. The School of Nursing for Women was dissolved in the same year, and an educational program that attracted both men and women operated until its closing in 1974 (University of Pennsylvania Health System, 2005c).

Student Life at the Pennsylvania Hospital School of Nursing for Men

I interviewed Luther Christman, PhD, RN, FAAN, and Claude Paoloni, RN, PhD, graduates of the Class of 1939, separately in 1998. Each was interviewed in his own home over a period of several hours on at least 2 separate days. Each had unique memories of his time as a student nurse, and the two interviewees seldom related the same information. Their stories did not conflict, but were uniquely their own.

There appeared to be two routes to admission to the school of nursing. Some men simply appeared at the hospital and were employed as assistants. The work involved 12-hour days, 6 days per week, for $15 per month, plus room, board, and laundry. When a class of students was planned, these men were then encouraged to apply for admission. Paoloni entered via this route, working at the Philadelphia Hospital in 1935 and being admitted to nursing in 1936. Paoloni stated that when school started, each student received a stipend of $10 per month for the first year, $15 per month for the second year, and $20 per month for the last six months of the third year, as well as room, board, and laundry.

Christman applied for admission to nursing upon graduation from high school. A Methodist minister who understood the unhappy circumstances of Christman's home life counseled Christman to enter nursing. He suggested that it might be the only way Christman could afford to continue his education, given his mother's animosity and the financial condition of the country during the Depression. Christman remembers a 2-day period of testing and interviews with Mr. Craig, other faculty members, and students. Part of the process included intelligence and personality testing, while a second part of the process included a lunch with Mr. Craig. At this time, the image of men in nursing was of concern to many inside and outside health care, so the purpose of the lunch was to explore the social graces possessed by the applicant. Christman recalled one student who passed all the tests with flying colors but was rejected because, during lunch with Mr. Craig, he buttered an entire slice of bread at once rather than breaking off smaller pieces and buttering the pieces as they were consumed.

The first and third years of the curriculum involved psychiatric nursing at the Hospital for Mental and Nervous Diseases. The second year involved an affiliation at the downtown hospital where the school for women was housed. Students received instruction in medical nursing, surgical nursing, urological nursing, operating room technique, and perhaps a little emergency nursing. They were not permitted to be taught or assigned in the areas of obstetrics and pediatrics and were not permitted access to the textbooks for those classes. However, when the men graduates took the nursing examinations for licensure they were required to pass the obstetric and pediatric exams. Both Paoloni and Christman remembered receiving textbooks from their fiancés, who were enrolled in nursing school in Philadelphia at the same time, so they could prepare for the exam.

Paoloni recalled being expelled from school midway through the program. He was working in the psychiatric unit and had escorted patients to the hospital ball park. The coach of the school's softball team was short of a player and ordered Paoloni to play rather than having to forfeit the game. Paoloni protested since he was supervising patients. The coach ordered him to play anyway and offered to supervise the patients for him. When the game was over, it was found that one of the patients had disappeared. Paoloni was convicted of dereliction of duty and was expelled. The coach denied any involvement in the case, but the assistant director of nursing was aware of what had really happened. The assistant director told Paoloni to go home, enjoy a short vacation, and apply for readmission in two weeks. Paoloni followed his directions, was reinstated, and subsequently graduated.

Christman, also, was almost expelled while working in the operating room. A urologist was doing a cystoscopy on a female patient and called for Christman to come into the room. When Christman got there, the physician invited him to look at the bladder tumor through the cystoscope. As Christman observed the tumor, the female supervisor walked in, noting Christman in a room with a female patient. She demanded that Christman be expelled from the school for unprofessional behavior. Christman also enjoyed a short vacation and was then quietly readmitted to the program.

Both men also remembered that they were required to bring tennis equipment and clothing to school as students. The image of men in nursing seemed to be the issue, and the belief at that time was that homosexual men would not play sports. So, by requiring sports in school, the school believed it would automatically eliminate any homosexual applicants (L. Christman & C. Paoloni, personal communication, 1998).

SUMMARY

Men and other minorities in nursing in the United States are seldom documented in the nursing literature. When men are mentioned, it is usually in passing and in a fashion that tends to marginalize them even more than the great silence. There were schools of nursing for men in the United States from the late 1880s until 1969. Their names and their precise number are probably lost to history. Sources document only some of these schools, yet there are still graduates of nursing schools for men in active nursing practice today. Very little is known about some of these schools. For example, there was a school for male nurses on Welfare Island, NY, which is said to have graduated about 140 men, most of whom went on to become physicians (J. Castille, personal communication, 1996). Also, Wilson (1997) reports that a school for men operated at St. Vincent's Hospital, New York, in about 1888. After that time, some schools of nursing for women created separate sections within their schools for men students when men were allowed to be admitted. Craig (1940) notes that in September 1939, four schools of nursing admitted only men, and 70 schools of nursing admitted both men and women, most of them in East Coast states, with the remainder of nursing schools admitting only women.

Men have continued to respond to the call to become nurses since the Middle Ages. Many of them responded by serving their countries through military service. Although men were denied admission to the military nurse corps until 1955, men nurses served in the armed forces during periods of conflict. During World War II, Paoloni was assigned as a corpsman and ran operating rooms while being paid and treated as an enlisted man. Christman was assigned to a nonmedical unit, even though nurses were in great demand and a draft of registered nurses was under consideration. Even though men were allowed to serve in the Army Nurse Corps as reserve officers in 1955, the Navy Nurse Corps refused to commission them until 1965, and the Air Force Nurse Corps limited men nurses to 300 slots initially.

The Vietnam War created a major dilemma for the military nurse corps. Consequently, by 1965, men nurses were authorized to apply for regular status and 3,000 men were drafted into the Army Nurse Corps. Many of the men drafted had served in Korea and had no draft obligation. Others had not functioned as registered nurses for years but had worked in other occupational fields. They had maintained their licenses as registered nurses and were recalled or called to active duty. Graduates of associate's degree programs in nursing were not eligible for commissioned status in the military nurse corps, but in 1965, these graduates were called to duty and commissioned as warrant officers. The first hospital staffed with registered nurses sent into Vietnam in 1962 was staffed by male Army Nurse Corps officers. Lt. Jerome (Jerry) Olmsted, a graduate of the Alexian Brothers Hospital School of Nursing Class of 1964, was killed in Vietnam when the fixed-wing airplane he was riding in for transport to a different assignment in was shot down during the Tet Offensive (Tranbarger, 1996). Olmstead's name is engraved on the Vietnam Memorial Wall on panel 31 E, but organized nursing continues to document only the eight women nurses who died in Vietnam. Also killed in the airplane crash was Kenneth Shoemaker, ANC, a certified registered nurse anesthetist. The Nurses Memorial within the Vietnam Memorial in Washington, DC, depicts only women nurses. Nowhere is there any reference to the men who served as registered nurses in Vietnam.

Men are again the focus of both concern and hope within nursing. The growing shortage of nurses and the escalating demand for nursing care cannot be met with the traditional White female applicants. History indicates that men can be recruited to nursing and most will serve with distinction when permitted to do so. The care of clients is not compromised in the process. The future of nursing will continue to be written by those brave and caring souls, of whatever gender and/or ethnicity, who deliver nursing services daily to clients throughout our health care system.

A Few Men Nurses of Distinction in the United States

L. Bissell Sanford, RN:

- Graduate of Mills Training School for Men, Bellevue, New York
- Appointed to New York State Board of Nurse Examiners in 1905
- First man to become a registered nurse in the United States
- Director of Mills Training Program

Leroy Craig, RN:

- Graduate of McLean Hospital, School of Nursing for Men
- Appointed director of nursing, Pennsylvania Hospital School of Nursing for Men
- Served as director until school closed in 1965
- Collaborated with Congresswoman Frances Paine Bolton to secure commissioned status for men in the Army Nurse Corps: this was achieved in 1955

E.W. Hearst, RN:

- Graduated from Mills Training School for Men, Bellevue, New York

- Appointed first director, Alexian Brothers Hospital School of Nursing, Chicago, 1898

Brother Maurice Wilson, CFA, RN:

- Graduated from the Alexian Brothers Hospital School of Nursing in 1952
- Appointed director of nursing, Alexian Brothers, Chicago, 1953
- Served until closing of school in 1969

Lawrence A. Sumler, RN:

- Graduated from Mills Training School for Men, Bellevue, New York, 1942
- First African American man to become a registered nurse in the United States

Edward Lyon, RN:

- First man to be commissioned a reserve officer in the Army Nurse Corps

Jerome Olmsted, RN:

- Graduated from the Alexian Brothers Hospital School of Nursing, Chicago, 1964
- Killed in Vietnam when the helicopter he was being transported in was shot down during the Tet Offensive, 1969

Joseph Barry, RN:

- Graduated from Mills Training School for Men, New York, 1954.
- Elected recording secretary, National Student Nurses Association (NSNA), 1954, becoming first man to hold office in NSNA

Michael Desjardins:

- Elected president of the National Student Nurses Association in 2001, the first man elected to that office

William Bester, RN, MS:

- Graduated from St. Scholastica College of Nursing, Duluth, MN

- Graduated from Madigan General Army Hospital, Anesthesia Program
- Received a master's degree in education, Catholic University, Washington, DC
- Appointed hospital commanding officer, Ft. Jackson, SC, the first nurse to hold this appointment; promoted to brigadier general and chief of the Army Nurse Corps, the first man to hold this position in the military (Tranbarger, 2001)

Luther Christman, RN:

- Graduated from the Pennsylvania Hospital School of Nursing for Men, Philadelphia, 1939
- Created Integration Model for Nursing Education and Service
- Founding dean, Rush College of Nursing, Chicago
- Cofounder, American Assembly for Men in Nursing
- First man elected to the American Academy of Nursing
- First man nominated for president of the American Nurses Association
- Named a "Living Legend" by the American Academy of Nursing
- Inducted into the Hall of Fame of the American Nurses Association, 2004; first man in the Hall of Fame
- Advocated for the commissioning of men registered nurses in the Armed Forces Nurse Corps during and after World War II
- Advocate for doctoral education and advanced practice for nurses

REFERENCES

Alexian Brothers. (2002). *Alumni Directory: Alexian Brothers Hospitals: Schools of nursing and radiologic technology, Chicago and St. Louis.* Chicago: Author.
Alexian Brothers. (2005a). *About the Brothers.* Retrieved March 14, 2005, from http://www.alexianbrothers.org/english/about/seal.html
Alexian Brothers. (2005b). *History: Alexian Brothers Hospital School of Nursing, Chicago, Illinois.* Retrieved March 14, 2005, from http://www.alexianbrothers.org/english/history/america/hist-nrs-chi.html
Alexian Brothers. (2005c). *History: Alexian Brothers Hospital School of Nursing: St. Louis, MO.* Retrieved March 14, 2005, from http://www.alexianbrothers.org/english/history/america/hist-nrs-stl.html
Bellevue Alumnae Association Collection. (2004). *Administrative history.* Retrieved May 25, 2005, from http://www.foundationnysnurses.org/collections/bellevuefa.htm
Craig, L. N. (1940). Opportunities for men nurses. *American Journal of Nursing, 40*(6), 666–670.

Kauffman, C. J. (1976). *Tamers of death: The history of the Alexian Brothers*. New York: Seabury Press.

New York State Board of Examiners of Registered Nurses. (1905). *Minutes of September 15, 1905*. Albany, NY: Author.

Pokorny, M. E. (1992). An historical perspective of confederate nursing during the Civil War, 1861–1865. *Nursing Research, 41*(1), 29.

Tranbarger, R. (1996). Honoring our veterans. *Interaction, 14*(4), 1, 3.

Tranbarger, R. (2001). B. G. William Bester, ANC, Chief, Army Nurse Corps. *Interaction, 18*(4), 1, 12.

University of Pennsylvania Health System. (2005a). Pennsylvania Hospital history: Historical timeline. Retrieved March 14, 2005, from http://www.uphs.upenn.edu/paharc/timeline/1751/

University of Pennsylvania Health System. (2005b). Pennsylvania Hospital history: Historical timeline. Retrieved March 14, 2005, from http://www.uphs.upenn.edu/paharc/timeline/1851/

University of Pennsylvania Health System. (2005c). Pennsylvania Hospital history: School of nursing for men. Retrieved March 14, 2005, from http://www.uphs.upenn.edu/paharc/timeline/1901/tline26.html

Whitman, W. (1865/1975). The wound dresser. In F. Murphy (Ed), *Walt Whitman: The Complete Poems* (pp. 333–336). New York: Penguin Books.

Wilson, B. (1997). Men in American nursing history. Retrieved July 4, 2005, from http://www.geocities.com/Athens/Forum/6011/sld003.htm

Curriculum and Faculty, Alexian Brothers School of Nursing, 1956–1959

Anatomy	Alan Antonik, BS
Chemistry	Alan Antonik, BS
Communicable Disease Nursing	Howard E. Kanous, RN, BSN
Diet Therapy	Margaret Phin, BS
Dermatological and Venereal Nursing	Virgil E. Guth, RN
Emergency Nursing	Rosalie Skowron, RN
English I	Lawrence A. Wallace, MA
Ethics	Rev. Clement Jagodzinski, MA
Ear, Eye, Nose, and Throat Diseases	Alfred Stonehill, MD
Gynecology	Jerome Weil, MD
Introduction to Medical Science	James P. Simonds, MD
Medical Nursing	Brother Lambert, CFA
Microbiology	Alan Antonik, BS
Nursing, Fundamentals of	Brother Cornelius, CFA
Nutrition	Marjorie Andrews, BS
Operating Room Technique	Robert Campbell, RN
Orthopedic Nursing	Howard E. Kanous, RN, BSN
Pharmacology I and II	Brother Dominick, CFA, RN, BS
Physiology	Alan Antonik, BS
Professional Adjustments I	Brother Maurice, CFA, RN, MA
Professional Adjustments II	Brother Maurice, CFA, RN, MA
Nursing History	Robert E. Briggs, RN
Psychology	Robert E. Briggs, RN
Religion I and II	Rev. Clement Jagodzinski, MA

Sociology	Robert E. Briggs, RN
Surgical Nursing	Howard E. Kanous, RN, BSN
Swimming	Arnold Cronin, RN
Urological Nursing	Virgil E. Guth, RN
Affiliations	
Maternity Nursing	Mercy Hospital, Chicago, IL
Pediatric Nursing	Children's Memorial Hospital, Chicago, IL
Psychiatry and Neurology	Alexian Brothers Hospital, St. Louis, MO
Tuberculosis Nursing	Municipal Tuberculosis Sanitarium, Chicago, IL

The American Assembly for Men in Nursing (AAMN): The First 30 Years as Reported in *Interaction*

Russell E . Tranbarger

INTRODUCTION

Nursing organizations have unique purposes and objectives that precipitate the need for their formation. In the early days of modern nursing, schools of nursing were established anywhere a hospital existed. In the late 19th century, when two doctors began to practice in the same town, often the first thing they did was start a hospital and organize a nursing program to staff it. In order to achieve standardization and consistency among the growing numbers of schools of nursing, the National League for Nursing was formed in 1893 (National League for Nursing, 2005). The American Nurses Association (ANA) was formed in 1897 (as the Nurses' Associated Alumnae of the United States and Canada), also to evaluate nursing curricula, as well as to support and advocate for graduates of nursing schools (Nursing World, 2005).

During the American Civil War, about half of the people who contracted to provide nursing to the Union soldiers were men. Perhaps the most famous of these was the poet Walt Whitman. One of his poems, "The Wound Dresser," tells about changing the dressing on a wounded soldier (Whitman, 1865/1975). However, by the dawn of the 20th century, the percentage of nurses who were men had fallen from approximately 50% to less than 1%, as the Nightingale model of nursing education and practice gained dominance (Miller, 1989). Men were discouraged from nursing, while at the same time physicians began to recognize that two standards of nursing care were quickly developing. Women patients received more expert care as women nurses gained nursing knowledge and skill, whereas the care of male patients was delegated to poorly trained, or often untrained, orderlies. Schools of nursing for men were set up to provide a more knowledgeable nurse to care for psychiatric patients and for men with urological problems. The Mills School of Nursing for Men at the Bellevue Hospital in New York was the first of these schools (Goodrich, n.d.). Chapter 2 in this book highlights the history of these early schools of nursing for men.

Discrimination against men in nursing continued unabated during the 20th century. Men nurses were denied admission to most nursing schools. They were not permitted to be commissioned in the Army Nurse Corps until 1955 and could not join the Navy Nurse Corps until 1965. The ANA denied membership to men nurses until 1930 (American Nurses Association, 1930). In 1940, the ANA established a men's interest group so that men could meet, share experiences, and address their needs (Casteel, 1996; R. Barry, personal communication, June 2005). However, many state associations did not allow men to join until the 1950s.

EARLY YEARS OF THE AAMN

In 1971, Steve Miller, a nurse, saw the need for an organization for men in nursing and formed a group of like-minded men in Michigan. The group grew in numbers and is reported to have had as many as 2,300 members. Luther Christman was invited to join the group and assist them with the development of the organization (L. Christman, personal communication, May 2005). Shortly thereafter, Miller decided to go to law school, and the organization floundered without his leadership.

In 1974, Christman convened a group of men nurses in Chicago, and the Men in Nursing in Michigan group was reorganized as the National Male Nurses Association. At this time, the percentage of American nurses who were men had increased, but only to about 3%. Thus, it is not surprising that the major purpose of the new organization was to foster the recruitment of more men, especially young men, into nursing ("More Men Needed in Nursing," 1982).

In 1981, The National Male Nurses Association was renamed the American Assembly for Men in Nursing (AAMN; "What the Assembly

Is About," 1989). In 1990, the objectives of the AAMN were described as follows:

> The objectives of the American Assembly for Men in Nursing are few and brief. We wholeheartedly encourage men, particularly young men, to become nurses and join together with other nurses in strengthening and humanizing health care for Americans. It is our goal to enhance the profession of nursing by increasing the visibility of men in the profession. ("The Objectives of AAMN," 1990)

Christman (1990) described the organization in this way:

> The American Assembly for Men in Nursing is primarily a caucus group to enable men in the nursing profession to have professional interchange, to develop social networks to facilitate communications of developments and innovation in the profession, and to assist in the major effort to unify the nursing profession.
>
> The benefit of membership comes from the free and open discussion of the professional issues in nursing seen from the viewpoint of being both a minority and men. The opportunity to have contact with potential mentors and/or behavioral models is enhanced. Furthermore, the visibility of the organization as it grows numerically will ease the way for effective recruitment of men into the nursing profession. A useful platform for better communication to the public about the nursing profession and its male membership is being created and developed. All these characteristics and benefits are beginning to emerge clearly. As the membership grows, more options for constructive action will become apparent.
>
> Membership is open to any nurse—male or female. The inclusion of both sexes in the organization will better enable the testing of ideations and concepts. A better dialogue between and among nurses can take place. (p. 1)

By this time, the AAMN had moved from the recruitment of men into nursing as its essential purpose to the goal of providing a forum for men in nursing to establish networking opportunities, identify potential mentors, and engage in professional issues and discussions from the perspectives of men and of men as a minority in nursing. Considerable emphasis was placed on the need to include women nurses in the organization's activities in order to ensure a dialogue among and between nurses of both genders.

It is most interesting that Christman (1990) stated that the AAMN could contribute to the effort to unify the profession. The period of the organization's origin and development coincided with the proposal by the ANA to move to the baccalaureate degree as the entry into nursing.

To say that the proposal was controversial in nursing would be an understatement! This issue continues to fragment the profession.

Other issues confronted the nursing profession during the 1980s and 1990s. The AAMN provided the voice of men nurses through resolutions and positions statements. The topics of these resolutions and statements include the following:

1. Gender equality in nursing education (adopted in 1984)
2. Opposition to registered care technicians and other assistive workers (adopted in 1989)
3. Statement on HIV in the health care setting (adopted in 1992)
4. Clinical assignments for male nursing students (adopted in 1993)
5. Cooperation between the AAMN and the ANA (adopted in 1994)
6. Use of gender-neutral language (adopted in 1996)

The full text of these resolutions and positions statements is given in Appendix A.

THE AAMN IN THE 21ST CENTURY

During the 1990s, the AAMN suffered some financial losses in its relationship with a management firm and due to declining membership. By 2002, the organization had recouped its financial losses and had built up a small savings fund. In addition, the organization had established the AAMN Foundation in 2000 in order to provide a tax-exempt vehicle to further its goals. In 2002, the board of directors of the AAMN appointed an ad hoc task force to develop a strategic plan for the organization. The general sense of the board seemed to be that the time was right for a renewal of the organization and for a push to take the AAMN to the next level.

In 2004, the AAMN members at the annual conference in Tucson, AZ, adopted revisions to the organization's mission, purposes, and objectives as proposed by the strategic planning task force. The new mission was stated as follows: "The primary mission of AAMN is to be the acknowledged national organization for men in nursing which influences national policy, research and education about men in nursing" (American Assembly for Men in Nursing [AAMN], 2005, p. 3). The purpose of the AAMN is to "provide a framework for nurses, as a group, to meet, to discuss, and influence factors which affect men as nurses" (AAMN, 2005, p. 3). The new objectives are to achieve the following:

1. Encourage men of all ages to become nurses and join together with all nurses in strengthening and humanizing health care.
2. Support men who are nurses to grow professionally and demonstrate to each other and to society the increasing contributions made by men within the nursing profession.
3. Advocate for continued research, education, and dissemination of information about men's health issues, men in nursing, and nursing knowledge at the local and national levels.
4. Support members' full participation in the nursing profession and its organizations, and use this Assembly for the limited objectives stated above. (AAMN, 2005, p. 3)

With these revisions, adopted in 2004, the organization boldly states its intent to be viewed as the national organization for men in nursing and commits itself to action in the areas of policy, research, and education regarding men in nursing and men's health. The organization continues to walk a fine line as an advocate for men to become nurses while fostering women as full members of the organization. Part of the value of the AAMN is its ability to provide a safe place for men and women nurses to engage in a full and open discussion of issues and a sharing of the differences in perspectives on issues based on gender.

In 2004, the AAMN Foundation received a grant from Johnson & Johnson that enabled the foundation to award the first nursing education scholarships designed specifically for men students. The first 10 such scholarships were awarded in 2005. The scholarships were awarded to men in both entry level and advanced nursing programs, selected from an applicant field of more than 150. The AAMN also recognizes men and women and organizations who have contributed significantly to the increased visibility and/or acceptance of men in nursing through various awards and through membership in the Society of Luther Christman Fellows. The society is a mechanism that raises funds for the foundation to continue to provide nursing scholarships and other projects in honor of Luther Christman, the founder of the AAMN and the first male inducted into the ANA's Hall of Fame.

Also in 2004, the AAMN redeveloped its presence on the Internet, making it easier to access organizational information and information related to men in nursing and to men's health. The Web site also provides a forum for men in nursing to discuss their experiences in nursing and to seek advice and support from other men and women who support men in nursing. The organization continues to sponsor annual conferences that provide researchers and others with opportunities to present their findings about men in nursing, men's health, and related issues in an atmosphere of respect and understanding. The AAMN newsletter, *Interaction,* provides a forum for the sharing of findings in print and is the only source for some research on these issues. *Interaction* has been available in the Cumulative Index to Nursing and Allied Health Literature (CINAHL) database since 1996.

EDUCATIONAL CONFERENCES

Since its earliest days, the AAMN has offered an annual educational conference. The conferences developed a tradition of focusing in one year on men's health issues and in the following year on issues of gender in nursing. Keynote conference speakers have been drawn from the ranks of national leaders, including Barbara Holtzclaw; Ada Sue Hinshaw; ANA President Beverly Malone; U.S. Senator Terry Sanford; Army Nurse Corps Chief Brigadier General William Bester; and Sigma Theta Tau International President Dan Pesut, to name just a few.

Conferences have been held in different parts of the country. Chicago has hosted more conferences than any other city, but the AAMN has developed a tradition of moving the conference location from north to south and east to west to equalize expenses, tap into the pockets of interested groups, and provide conference attendees with an opportunity to visit places of interest. The AAMN has provided nursing students with either reduced rates or free conference registration in order to further the organization's objectives. Of important note, the educational conferences in themselves have made, and continue to make, a unique contribution to nursing, since the AAMN remains the only nursing organization to focus on issues of men's health.

SUMMARY

The AAMN has weathered many challenges during its existence. Its membership has dropped from more than 1,000 to less than 50 and has recovered once more. The organization has divided itself over issues of gender orientation, educational preparation for entry into nursing, and other issues that have caused great angst in the nursing profession generally. Some elected AAMN officers have disappeared after their election, and some have taken membership mailing lists and perhaps organizational funds with them. Yet, men in nursing continue to grow in numbers and in visibility. The AAMN continues to present the existence and voices of men in nursing to the public as well as to nursing itself. The AAMN has joined the Nursing Organization Liaison Forum (NOLF) with the ANA, presented lectures on issues of men's health and issues unique to men in nursing, monitored actions affecting men in nursing, and established a legal fund to provide assistance to men fighting battles over discrimination against them in nursing. Individual members of the AAMN have provided uncounted contributions to the profession, including authoring numerous articles and letters to editors addressing men's health and men in nursing. The AAMN remains the only nursing organization that speaks for men in nursing and the only nursing organization to advocate on issues of men's health. Today, the public views men in nursing more positively than in previous decades, and the media increasingly deal with men in nursing not as oddities but as men working in just one more field they choose. Today, acceptance of men as nurses is seldom a workplace issue. As the 21st century unfolds, the future of men in nursing looks very promising and the AAMN remains the best kept secret in nursing!

REFERENCES

American Assembly for Men in Nursing (AAMN). (2005). *Bylaws.* Latham, NY: Author.

American Nurses Association. (1930). *Proceedings of the twenty-seventh convention of the American Nurses Association.* Silver Spring, MD: Author.

Casteel, J. (1996). A brief chronology of the history of men in nursing. *Interaction, 14*(2), 10.

Christman, L. (1990). The Assembly's mission. *Interaction, 7*(3), 1.

Goodrich, A. W. (n.d.). Bellevue Alumnae Association Collection, box 2, series 1, Bellevue Hospital, New York.

Miller, T. (1989). History and socialization of men in nursing. *Interaction, 6*(2), 2.

More men needed in nursing. (1982). *Interaction, 1*(3), 1–2.

National League for Nursing. (2005). *History of the National League for Nursing (NLN) supporting nursing education for over a century.* Retrieved June 18, 2005, from http://www.nln.org/aboutnln/info-history.htm

Nursing World. (2005). *Voices from the past, visions of the future.* Retrieved June 18, 2005, from http://www.nursingworld.org/centenn/#exhibit

The objectives of AAMN. (1990). *Interaction, 7*(4), 1.

What the Assembly is about. (1989). *Interaction, 6*(2), 1.

Whitman, W. (1865/1975). The wound dresser. In F. Murphy (Ed.), *Walt Whitman: The complete poems* (pp. 333–336). New York: Penguin Books.

APPENDIX A

Resolutions and Position Statements of the American Assembly for Men in Nursing

1. POSITION STATEMENT: GENDER EQUALITY IN NURSING EDUCATION

Every professional nurse position and every nursing educational opportunity shall be equally available to those meeting the entry qualifications regardless of gender. (Adopted December 1983, and circulated to the membership for reactions.) *Interaction* (1984), *3*(1).

2. RESOLUTION: RESOLUTION AGAINST REGISTERED CARE TECHNICIAN (RCT) AND OTHER CATEGORIES OF ASSISTIVE WORKERS (as adopted at the 1989 annual meeting)

WHEREAS, the RCT has been proposed as a new care giver in the hospital by the American Medical Association, specifically targeting men and minorities, and the educational curriculum has not yet been designed and many regulatory, supervisory, and liability questions have not yet been answered, and the proposed duties are already within the range of duties of existing nursing personnel and would cost hospitals and taxpayers more money, and high school graduates with only 2–18 months training would be carrying out "medical protocols" at the bedside where mistakes can least be afforded, and men and other minorities in nursing will experience limited career mobility on entering as an RCT and already have methods of entry into the nursing profession, BE IT RESOLVED THAT, AAMN supports the American Nurses Association and other professional organizations in their opposition to the RCT, and AAMN will designate a monetary sum to be used in opposing the RCT, and AAMN will monitor and update its members via Interaction concerning RCT political activity, and AAMN will write selected Congressmen and presidents of medical and nursing organizations, as well as encourage individuals to write their congressmen, and finally, AAMN will educate nursing and medical personnel, as well as the general public, about the continual need for more registered nurses to supply the increasing needs of hospitals. *Interaction* (1990), 7(2).

3. RESOLUTION: HIV IN THE HEALTH CARE SETTING WHEREAS AAMN is committed to the prevention of HIV transmission, and

    a. There is public concern about the risk of HIV transmission from health care providers, and
    b. There are calls for restrictions on the practice of competent health care providers which would limit access to health care, and
    c. Scientific evidence supports universal precautions, used consistently, as providing the most comprehensive protection for consumers and health care providers,

THEREFORE BE IT RESOLVED THAT AAMN

a. Affirm its position in support of the public's protection from HIV infections, and
b. Endorse universal precautions, including adequate disinfection techniques, as the most effective protection for consumers and providers in all health care settings, and
c. Vigorously opposes mandatory testing of nurses and other health care providers, and
d. Strongly encourages those infected with HIV to act responsibly and professionally in their practices to ensure the safety of their clients/patients, and
e. Opposes the development of lists of exposure-prone procedures, and
f. Call for continuing research and development of safer equipment, improved universal precaution techniques, and full access to safer equipment in all health care settings.

IMPLEMENTATION: AAMN WILL

a. Publish this resolution in *Interaction*.
b. Communicate this resolution to appropriate organizations engaged in the provision of health care.
c. Communicate its position to the CDC.
d. Provide an update of the status of this issue to the members at the 1992 Annual Meeting in Atlanta. *Interaction* (1992), 10(1), 2.

4. RESOLUTION: RESOLUTION ON CLINICAL ASSIGNMENTS FOR MALE NURSING STUDENTS (December 3, 1993)

The American Assembly for Men in Nursing is concerned to receive reports that in some schools of nursing, and in some clinical facilities, a student's gender or race may constitute a bar to clinical expertise.

WHEREAS,

a.   The AAMN regards bias associated with gender or race as inherently discriminatory in character and views the consequences of such discrimination as serious and unacceptable for students whose practice is thus restricted. Such restriction may also lead to deficiencies in necessary clinical experiences.
b.   The existence of bias toward gender or race in nursing education calls into question the ethical integrity of the nursing profession itself, therefore

BE IT RESOLVED,

The American Assembly for Men in Nursing categorically opposes any consideration of gender or race as determinants for the clinical assignments of students in nursing. *Interaction* (1994), *12*(1), 5.

5.   RESOLUTION: COOPERATION BETWEEN THE AAMN and THE ANA

WHEREAS,

a.   The American Assembly for Men in Nursing has since 1974 promoted the recruitment of men into the nursing profession, and
b.   The American Assembly for Men in Nursing has encouraged and supported the professional growth of men in the nursing profession, and
c.   An objective of the American Assembly for Men in Nursing reads "this Assembly intends that its members be full participants in the nursing profession and its professional associations and use this Assembly for its limited objectives," and
d.   The American Nurses Association, the professional association for all nurses in the United States, had a Men Nurses Section from 1940–1952, and
e.   Both these distinguished organizations for professional nurses can accomplish their respective and joint goals better together, then therefore

BE IT RESOLVED,

The American Assembly for Men in Nursing seek the highest level of cooperation with the American Nurses Association to recruit and retain men nurses and encourage active participation in both organizations by, and through, their member nurses. *Interaction* (1994), *12*(1), 5.

6. POSITION STATEMENT: THE USE OF GENDER NEUTRAL
    LANGUAGE IN THE NURSING LITERATURE

The American Assembly for Men in Nursing (AAMN) recognizes that
there is an editorial tendency in nursing specialty journals to rely on the
gender specific pronoun "she" when referring to the nurse. While nursing
education has taken the position that writing should be gender neutral,
this is not the case with articles in the literature.

PURPOSE

The purpose of this position statement is to delineate AAMN's beliefs
about the appropriate use and gender reference for the word "nurse."

BACKGROUND

Morse (1995) has called for the use of "inclusive language" that is not
gender specific and respects the individual worth, dignity, and integrity of
all human beings. This is consistent with the feminist pedagogy that insists
on equal treatment for genders. Such changes have been incorporated for
the most part in the curricula in academia and thus it is incumbent that
we remind publishers to be aware of what they are publishing. Nursing
literature that is true to its source is literature that is inclusive. Thus, the
language and subject matter should be critically reviewed for inclusiveness. Exclusive language reinforces biased thinking. If gender references
are so dichotomous, then we perpetuate these stereotypes in our profession. Bias can and should be avoided by the use of "inclusive language."
Such a stance is not unique. Specific instruction is given by the American Psychological Association (1994) that "constructions that might imply bias against persons on the basis of gender, sexual orientation, race,
ethnic group, disability or age should be avoided" (p. 46).

Recently, there has been discussion of the tendency of publications
to think of the "bad nurse" as a male (Coffey, 1996; Smith & Hughes,
1996; Sprouse, 1996a, 1996b). This is the exception to the usual rule of
referring to nurses as "she." It indicates that the problem in the literature
is not resolved.

Caring is a universal, androgynous trait. Good nurses must be
independent, able to solve problems and serve as patient advocates (traits
usually culturally attributed to males) as well as to be nurturing and
sympathetic (traits culturally assigned to females). Nursing is concerned
with the well-being of the total person and is not gender biased toward

patients. For this reason, good nursing requires that the most qualified nurse (male or female) is designated for patient care. This sentiment is echoed in the position of the Association of Women's Health, Obstetric, and Neonatal Nurses (1995), which states that "AWOHNN believes that all women's health, obstetric, and neonatal clients have the right to quality care provided by a clinically competent, professional nurse. Furthermore, AWOHNN believes that nurses, regardless of gender, should be employed in women's health, obstetric, and neonatal nursing based on their ability to provide care to the clients."

CONCLUSION

As an organization, the AAMN is committed to both the science of nursing and the fair treatment of individuals and groups. Therefore, it supports the following:

a. The effort of nursing leaders to require publishers to pay attention to professional language in their editorial review of publishable material.
b. The education of editorial staff to use inclusive language in nursing publications.

REFERENCES

American Psychological Association. (1994). *Publication manual of the American Psychological Association* (4th ed.). Washington, DC: Author.

Association for Women's Health, Obstetric, and Neonatal Nurses (AWOHNN). (1995). *Position statement: Gender as a qualification requirement for nursing positions in women's health, obstetric, and neonatal nursing.* Washington, DC: Author.

Coffey, C. (1996). Response to re-entry (Letter to the editor). *American Journal of Nursing, 96*(4), 20.

Morse, G. G. (1995). Reframing women's health in nursing education: A feminist approach. *Nursing Outlook, 43*(6), 273–277.

Smith, L. L., & Hughes, T. L. (1996). Re-entry: When a chemically dependent colleague returns to work. *American Journal of Nursing, 96*(2), 32–37.

Sprouse, D. (1996a). Message from the president. *Interaction, 14*(3), 1–2, 4.

Sprouse, D. (1996b). Message from the president. *Interaction, 14*(4), 6–7.

Presidents of the AAMN

Ed Halloran	1982–1984
Fred Farley	1984–1986
Frederick May	1986–1988
Lawrence J. Voyten	1988–1990
Terrill L. Stumpf	1990–1992
Lee Cohen	1992–1994
David Sprouse	1994–1996
J. Keenan Castille	1996*
Robert Schaffner	1997–1998
David Sprouse	1998–2000
Russell E. Tranbarger	2000–2004
Jim Raper	2004–

*Served less than 12 months

APPENDIX C

Keynote Speakers at AAMN Educational Conferences*

1981	Barbara Holtzclaw, PhD, RN, FAAN
1984	Jerome Lysaught
1986	Beverly Huckman
1987	Stanley Lesse, MD
1988	E. Ronald Wright, PhD
1989	Ada Sue Hinshaw, PhD, RN, FAAN
1990	Mary K. Wakefield, PhD, RN
1992	Nicholas A. Cummings, PhD (President, National Academies of Practice)
1993	Barbara Holtzclaw, PhD, RN, FAAN
1994	Warren Farrell, PhD (Author, *The Myth of Male Power: The Liberated Male*)
1995	Terry Sanford (former U.S. Senator, Governor, NC)
1997	James Harris, DNS, RN
1998	Marie O'Toole, EdD, RN, CRRN
1999	Beverly Malone, PhD, RN, FAAN (President, ANA)
2000	Greta Cammermeyer, PhD, RN
2001	Brigadier General William Bester, Chief, Army Nurse Corps
2002	Daniel Pesut, PhD, RN, FAAN
2003	Will Courtenay, PhD, LCSW (Director, Men's Health Consulting)
2004	Larry Purnell, PhD, RN, FAAN
2006	Edward Thompson, PhD (Director, Gerontology Studies Program, College of the Holy Cross)

*Note: Educational conferences with keynote speakers have not been offered every year.

CHAPTER FOUR

Army Nursing: A Personal Biography

William T. Bester

INTRODUCTION

It's been 31 years since I graduated from my baccalaureate nursing program at a small Catholic college, the College of St. Scholastica, in my hometown of Duluth, Minnesota. During these 31 years, I have been asked on numerous occasions, "If you had it to do all over again, would you choose nursing as a career?" I've always been able to answer that question with an unhesitating "Yes." Nursing has afforded me more opportunity, more diversity of professional experiences, and more job satisfaction than I could ever imagine being equaled by any other professional endeavor.

With the exception of this past year, my entire nursing career has been spent providing care to our American soldiers, their family members, and our retired military men and women. Until June 2004, I served as a proud member of the Army Nurse Corps. This past year has taken me into a new professional environment—that of academia. This new opportunity is currently providing me the chance to give something back to the profession by helping to educate the next generation of clinical nurses, nursing leaders, and nursing scholars.

My 30 years in the Army Nurse Corps (ANC) gave me the opportunity to practice within an organization that, from a gender perspective, is very different our profession as a whole. According to the ANC Branch at the U.S. Army Personnel Command, the percentage of men in the ANC is currently 35.48%, compared to approximately 6% of male nurses in the civilian nursing workforce. During my four years as chief of the ANC,

I was frequently asked why so many men have chosen to practice nursing in the Army. I don't believe this question has a single simple answer. Rather, I believe the high percentage of men in military nursing is due to a number of factors, including educational opportunities, leadership training, service to our nation; salary, health care, retirement benefits, and career-long opportunities for professional advancement and formalized specialty nursing courses. This chapter will look first at the history of male nurses within the ANC and will then focus on some of the positive factors identified above as they relate to my personal and professional opportunities over the past three decades.

HISTORICAL ESTABLISHMENT OF GENDER EQUALITY IN MILITARY NURSING

According to Major Charlotte Scott, ANC historian at the Office of Medical History within the Army's Surgeon General's Office, military nursing in the United States dates back to the American Revolution (C. Scott, personal communication, May 13, 2005). Inadequate help in caring for sick and wounded soldiers during this conflict often forced military commanders to pull soldiers from the front lines to provide care to those in need. Although these "providers" were not nurses in the formal sense of the word, the need to provide care to the sick and wounded was clear.

During the Civil War, the majority of nurses were female volunteers (C. Scott, personal communication, May 13, 2005). However, the need for larger numbers of individuals to care for the sick and the injured resulted in the establishment of the Hospital Corps by the Army's surgeon general. This was a corps of enlisted male soldiers who were trained in providing care to the wounded. During the Spanish-American War of 1898, most of the nursing care continued to be provided by female volunteers. However, male contract nurses were employed, and some that died were buried in Arlington National Cemetery (*Proud to Serve,* n.d.). On September 22, 1931, Edmund Kirby wrote a letter to the surgeon general asking for information regarding the number of male contract nurses employed during the period of the Spanish-American War (C. Scott, personal communication, May 13, 2005). In response to Mr. Kirby's request, Colonel J. B. Higgins replied that "633 male contract nurses were employed during the Spanish-American War" (copy of letter dated September 29, 1931, C. Scott, personal communication, May 13, 2005).

As a result of the outstanding performance of professional nursing personnel during the Spanish-American War and the identified need for nursing support in future conflicts, a bill was introduced to Congress in

1901 to establish a permanent Army Nurse Corps. On February 2, 1901, the Army Nurse Corps (ANC) became a permanent corps of the Army Medical Department under the Army Reorganization Act (31 Stat. 753) (*Proud to Serve*, n.d.). Although this was the formal beginning of the ANC, it was a corps limited to female members only. It would be some 54 years later before men would be allowed to obtain commissions as officers in the corps.

The years between 1901 and 1955 witnessed numerous attempts by a multitude of individuals to open membership in the ANC to male nurses. A great deal of resistance to these attempts to achieve gender equality persisted. Major William Terriberry, MD, addressed the issue of men in nursing and stated that "the lack of male nurses in the United States is due to the lack of a demand for them. In hospitals there is a small need for them now, and in the future this need will decrease" (Terriberry, 1908, p. 449).

During World War I, male nurses were not allowed to work as registered nurses but instead filled orderly positions in Army hospitals (*Proud to Serve*, n.d.; C. Scott, personal communication, May 13, 2005). A letter to U.S. Representative Charles B. Smith (1918) regarding this gender inequity within the Army system was sent by a Mr. Prince, a registered nurse working as an orderly in an Army hospital in France. He stated in his letter that "There are attached to the Buffalo B. H. #23 seven male nurses, men who have practiced such in civil life and hold state diplomas allowing them such rights; here we receive no recognition whatever, are classed as orderlies and paid about one half the salary of a female nurse." He went on to say that "The course of training is exactly the same for a male nurse as a female and what we ask, we feel perfectly justified in doing so, is equal classification both in rank and salary" (copy of letter dated April 13, 1918, National Archives, Record Group 112, Surgeon General's Office).

During World War II, male nurses continued to be barred from receiving commissions in the ANC. In a letter written to the editors of the *American Journal of Nursing*, H. R. Musser (1941) comments that

> In all states, registration is granted men only upon successful completion of a recognized course in nursing and passing of state board examinations. Nurse examiners have established these standards to ensure the registration of qualified nurses. Surely, such standardization should lead to professional equality in governmental rankings, equality meaning a standardized basic rating for all nurses, regardless of sex. (p. 1449)

In May 1942, the American Nurses Association's House of Delegates sent a letter to the surgeons general of the Army and Navy requesting that graduate, registered professional male nurses be given the opportunity to serve as nurses in the armed forces (American Nurses Association, 1942). In the same year, the American Hospital Association adopted the following resolution:

> That the Board of Trustees has endorsed the recommendation that graduate male nurses should be given the same status in the Army as graduate female nurses and that this resolution be sent to the Surgeons Generals of the Army, Navy, and the US Public Health Service. (American Nurses Association, 1942, p. 9)

In spite of both personal efforts and professional organizational requests to allow male nurses to serve in the armed forces of the United States, resistance continued. John Martyn, administrative assistant in the Office of the Chief of Staff in the War Department, wrote the following to U.S. Representative J. Hardin Peterson on January 17, 1945:

> The Surgeon General advises me that the question of using male nurses has been carefully considered, and it has been definitely concluded that male nurses are not desired for use as officers in the Army Nurse Corps. (copy of letter provided by C. Scott, personal communication, May 13, 2005)

A letter dated July 28, 1948, from Ethel Prince, representing the New York State Nurses Association, to U.S. Representative Emanuel Cellar (1948) argued that "Now is the time to make the necessary change in the law to admit male nurses to the Army Nurse Corps" (copy of letter provided by C. Scott, personal communication, May 13, 2005).

Support for male nurses to be allowed to join the Army Nurse Corps continued to grow. On August 10, 1950, U.S. Representative Frances P. Bolton (R-OH) introduced legislation to the 81st Congress (H.R. 9398) providing for the appointment of male citizens as nurses in the Army, Navy, and Air Force (*Proud to Serve,* n.d.). However, it would take this legislation some 5 more years before it would be passed into law. During those 5 years, much debate and some significant resistance continued.

In early 1950, just prior to Representative Bolton's proposed legislation, the chief of the Army Nurse Corps, Colonel Mary G. Phillips, sent out a letter to her senior nursing officers requesting their opinions regarding the commissioning of male nurses in the ANC. The responses she received clearly spell out the reluctance on the part of a number of senior ANC officers. The following responses were sent back to Colonel Phillips in early 1950:

Nursing the sick is definitely a woman's prerogative and even though the majority of patients in the Army are men, women nurses are more acceptable and adaptable from the professional and also personal angle. (LTC Elsie Schneider, Letterman General Hospital, San Francisco, CA; copy of letter dated January 26, 1950, provided by C. Scott, May 13, 2005)

After consulting the Commanding Officer, Executive Officer, Assistant Chief Nurse, and Nursing Supervisors, the opinion seems to be that we would have many problems arising as a result of commissioning male nurses in the Army Nurse Corps. One problem would be the attitude of male officers serving under the command and leadership of female officers ... it is not felt that male officers would be satisfied, happy or cooperative in serving under this authority. (Maj. Mabel Stott, William Beaumont General Hospital, El Paso, TX; copy of letter dated January 23, 1950, provided by C. Scott, May 13, 2005)

It is my opinion, therefore, that it would be extremely unwise to open the Nursing Corps to men nurses at this time. (LTC Ida Danielson, Army Medical Center, Washington, DC; copy of letter dated January 18, 1950, provided by C. Scott, May 13, 2005)

Personally I prefer that we do not have male nurses, but if Congress authorizes their admission I hope that the number allotted in the Corps will be in proportion to the entire civilian registered nurse population. (LTC Elizabeth Fitch, Headquarters Fifth Army, Chicago, IL; copy of letter dated January 12, 1950, provided by C. Scott, May 12, 2005)

I am sure it [the proposed legislation] is something we have all hoped would never really come up.... I personally do not believe we are ready to accept male nurses into the Army Nurse Corps and hope it will not come before this Congress. (LTC Katharine Jolliffe, Headquarters Third Army, Atlanta, GA; copy of letter dated January 9, 1950, provided by C. Scott, May 13, 2005)

In contrast, however, in a letter addressed to Representative Bolton in July 1950 (a month prior to the legislation being introduced), Major General R. W. Bliss, the Army surgeon general, stated that "I would not be personally opposed to such legislation" (copy of letter dated July 24, 1950, provided by C. Scott, May 13, 2005). A view opposing that of the surgeon general was voiced in October 1950 when Secretary of the Army Frank Pace Jr. sent a letter to the Honorable Carl Vinson, chairman of the Committee on Armed Services in the House of Representatives. In the letter, Pace declared that

It is believed that enactment of HR 9398 would impose administrative and legislative requirements upon the Department of Defense that would be unnecessarily burdensome. In view of the above comments, the Department of Defense is opposed to the enactment of HR 9398. (copy of letter dated October 5, 1950, provided by C. Scott, May 13, 2005)

The following year, 1951, a high-level Army Medical Department meeting was held to discuss the appointment and utilization policies of male nurses. In a memorandum for the record, LTC Katherine Bultz, ANC, stated that General Robinson, MD, the chief of the Personnel Division, queried the following individuals: Colonel Bowers, the chief of Surgical Services; Colonel Weir, representative from Medical Consultants; Colonel Merchant, a surgical consultant; Colonel Simmons, from Procurement; Colonel John Caldwell, Psychiatry; and Colonel Gingles, Personnel. With the exception of Colonel Gingles, all of the other men present thought the Army should accept male nurses in the ANC. It is interesting to note that Colonel Gingles, who opposed male nurses in the ANC, was quoted as saying that "I had no good reason, but I didn't think they should be part of the Corps." On the basis of these cumulative comments, General Robinson stated that a letter would be written and sent to the medical policy board that the surgeon general of the Army would go on record as not opposing the legislation (copy of memorandum dated January 23, 1951, provided by C. Scott, May 13, 2005).

The next four years were spent discussing, debating, and forwarding legislation, all in an attempt to move the commissioning of male nurses into the ANC closer to becoming a reality. Ultimately, on August 9, 1955, President Dwight D. Eisenhower signed Public Law 294, authorizing the commissioning of male nurses in the U.S. Army Reserve for assignment to the ANC (Craig, 1956; *Proud to Serve*, n.d.). After 54 years of debate and gender inequity, Edward L. T. Lyon, a nurse anesthetist from Kings Park, NY, was commissioned as a second lieutenant and became the first man to receive a commission in the ANC on October 6, 1955. Four days later, 2LT Edward Lyon entered active duty as an ANC officer (Boivin, 2002; *Proud to Serve*, n.d.).

Since that monumental day in 1955, the number of male nurses within the ANC has continued to grow to its present-day strength of over 1,100 male nurses serving on active duty in our Army. The groundbreaking work that those previously mentioned individuals accomplished, along with the persistent cry for gender equality by a number of professional nursing organizations, has allowed individuals such as myself and hundreds of other men to achieve professional success in our military.

However, the legislation that was passed simply provided the framework for the opportunity to be successful. Individual success, however, is almost always directly attributable to dedicated, caring, and professional individuals who ensure that the next generation of nursing professionals receives the teaching, the mentoring, the support, and the guidance to position them for success. My story is no different. I was blessed with outstanding mentors and teachers, who took a personal interest in assisting me to achieve the next level of professional advancement. Any success I have achieved during my professional military nursing career is directly attributable to these outstanding individuals.

MY PROFESSIONAL JOURNEY

My path in nursing actually began when I was enrolled as an accounting major at the University of Minnesota–Duluth. I had been in school for over two years, had changed majors three times, and was having difficulty finding a profession that truly excited me. Fortunately, I took a trip to a career counselor's office. I was given some aptitude tests and was told that I had scored well in the sciences and that the health care field might afford me some opportunities. I soon learned about the field of nurse anesthesia, spent some time at a local hospital visiting with nurse anesthetists, and then decided that nurse anesthesia was the professional path I wanted to pursue. I enrolled in a four-year program at the College of St. Scholastica (CSS) in Duluth. Since CSS was a private college, the tuition fees were significantly higher than I had been paying previously. I was the oldest of seven children and couldn't expect my parents to provide any financial assistance. One day, while walking the halls of CSS, I was approached by an Army recruiter and told about a program that paid tuition, books, and a monthly stipend for a payback of 3 years' service in the ANC upon graduation. I applied for the program at the end of my sophomore year in nursing school, was accepted for my junior and senior years, and started my journey down the road of Army nursing.

There were 55 students in our nursing class, 11 of whom were male. So, very early on in my nursing experience I was accustomed to seeing men in nursing. However, men were visibly nonexistent in teaching roles at the nursing school. Therefore, I had no male role models. The instructors we had at CSS, however, were excellent. I remember many to this day. One instructor in particular had a very strong influence on me. She was a no-nonsense, articulate, and extremely intelligent nurse. I learned much from her, but the one thing I remember most is a comment she made early on in my course of instruction. She said, "No matter what professional track you pursue in nursing, it is first and foremost extremely important that you develop strong clinical nursing skills." This made a significant impression on me. Following graduation, my primary focus was to seek out the type of clinical experiences I would need in order to develop these strong clinical skills.

My first two assignments in the Army included staff nurse positions on a multiservice surgical ward, a post-anesthesia care unit, and a combined medical/surgical intensive care unit. As a new graduate nurse, I was intimidated by the idea of caring for critically ill patients who were on ventilators, on dialysis machines, or connected to a variety of items of invasive monitoring equipment at the bedside. Fortunately for me, we had a team of very seasoned nurses who were willing to take the time to teach, train, and mentor each new graduate nurse. They personally helped me grow from a new graduate nurse to a highly effective critical care nurse. Of course, this didn't happen overnight. But through their continued persistence, I was able to elevate my clinical skills far beyond my imagination. It is interesting to note that all of my mentors and teachers during this phase of my nursing career were female.

In 1977, I entered the field of nurse anesthesia by attending the Army's Nurse Anesthesia Program. During my training and in the months immediately following my graduation, I was fortunate, once again, to be surrounded by individuals who were interested in elevating my skill level. This time, most of my mentors and teachers were male, and I have kept lifelong relationships with many of them. Without the caring and compassionate leadership and training I received early on in my career, I doubt very much that I would have been able to develop the sound clinical nursing skills that I attained. Those who mentored and taught me certainly affected my ability to achieve other professional successes. In fact, I often wonder if I would have remained in nursing without their guidance.

While assigned as a nurse anesthetist at Ft. Sill, OK, I was deployed to Ft. Chaffee, AR, as the sole anesthesia provider for the Cuban Refugee Operation. This experience of working in an environment totally different from my accustomed daily working environment sparked my interest in pursuing other nursing experiences outside the doors of the operating room. Because the Army had trained me in nurse anesthesia, I thought that they would not support me in pursuing other specialties. Therefore, I submitted the appropriate paperwork to leave the Army, in order to pursue opportunities as a civilian.

It was at this time that I appreciated the wisdom of my father, who had always said that timing was everything. When the paperwork requesting my discharge hit the desk of my director of nursing, she immediately asked me if she could hold the paperwork in her office for a couple of weeks. A visiting senior officer was scheduled to visit our installation soon, and she wanted me to talk with him before forwarding any paperwork to Washington, DC. When I met with the officer, I found him to be a very sincere, soft-spoken, and experienced officer who had also thought about leaving anesthesia for other opportunities in nursing. After discussing this issue with both him and my director of nursing, I made the decision to remain on active duty.

I've often looked back on this fortunate sequence of events and remain thankful to this day for these two individuals who cared so much about my personal and professional career choices. The timing of my encounter with these two individuals in my life at that point in time changed the course of my career path forever.

Enthused with my new journey, I asked for, and received, my first position out of anesthesia, as chief nurse of a combat support hospital. The chief nurse is primarily responsible for the medical training of all enlisted personnel, the coordination of training for the professional staff (i.e., nurses and physicians) who will deploy with the hospital, and the maintenance of and training with the medical equipment within the combat support hospital structure. Because the nurse anesthesia program was not a master's level program, some of my senior mentors recommended that I apply for graduate school following my assignment as chief nurse. This pursuit was possible, as the ANC funds approximately 100 nurses a year to pursue either a master's or a doctoral degree. Besides paying tuition and books, the ANC also continues to pay one's full salary. I applied for graduate education and was selected to enroll in a master's degree program at the Catholic University of America in Washington, DC.

Following my graduation, I was assigned to work as an instructor at the Academy of Health Sciences. During my tenure, I taught in our 1-year licensed practical nurse course, our nurse anesthesia program, and our officer advanced course. The positive experiences I gained during the 3 years at the academy, I believe, greatly influenced my decision to take a faculty position upon my eventual retirement from the ANC. My next assignment took me to Chicago, where I managed a 12-state nurse recruiting effort. Although I was not terribly excited about moving to this position, my senior assignments officer assured me that the experience I would gain managing personnel resources in such a large geographic area, coupled with the knowledge I would obtain regarding recruitment and retention issues, would pay big dividends for me in the long term. She was absolutely right. One of the largest issues we dealt with during my eventual tenure as chief of the ANC was the challenge of the national nursing shortage and the importance of an equally strong focus on both recruitment and retention. My experience in the late 1980s proved to be very helpful to me in the early 21st century.

My next assignment took me to the Washington, DC, area where I served as a personnel management officer, managing approximately

800 ANC officers' careers. I was responsible for ensuring that each officer attended the schools he or she needed, both military and civilian. In addition, I had the responsibility of the worldwide staffing and assignment of all the community health nurses, operating room nurses, and nurse anesthetists in the ANC. Again, this personnel experience proved extremely beneficial to me later on in my career.

My next assignment was at a small community hospital in Indianapolis as the director of nursing. The hospital was slated for closure. Consequently, a significant amount of my time was spent readying the staff, the community, and the physical structure for the impending closure, and preparing personnel for the transition to civilian health care. I feel the hospital closure was highly successful due, in part, to the work of some outstanding senior nurse leaders. I once had a boss who told me that one of the smartest things you can do as a leader is to surround yourself with people who are enthusiastic and intelligent. I was blessed to have those types of individuals surrounding me in Indianapolis.

With the impending closure, the ANC moved me to a new director of nursing position at Ft. Leavenworth, KS. However, my tenure in Kansas was short. I was promoted to colonel and was soon notified that I would be moving to Germany to become the director of nursing at the U.S. Army Hospital in Würzburg. Although I was truly enjoying my position at Ft. Leavenworth and was not anxious to move so soon, my career assignment branch felt that the position in Germany was necessary for me, as it was an advancement to a full colonel's position.

In addition to my duties as the director of nursing in Germany, I was also designated as the chief nurse of the 67th Combat Support Hospital (CSH), a "go to war" hospital available for deployment, anywhere it was needed, on short notice. Approximately 18 months after my arrival, the 67th CSH was alerted to deploy to the Balkans in support of the peace-enforcing mission, "Operation Joint Endeavor." Although my primary role was that of chief nurse of the combat support hospital, I was also selected to lead the advanced party into Hungary. We deployed on less than 24 hours' notice, 2 weeks before Christmas 1995. We transported both the hospital and our personnel by rail and arrived 2 days later at an old Russian airfield outside the small town of Taszar, Hungary. Our team immediately began to set up the hospital upon arrival. We needed to be fully operational in a matter of 24–48 hours in order for us to care for the 20,000 plus soldiers scheduled to start arriving in the next few days, as we would be the only American medical facility at that point in time in the area of Hungary, Croatia, and Bosnia. As our team of enlisted soldiers, physicians, nurses, and other professional health care personnel worked well into the night to complete the construction of the hospital structure, we were visited by the corps commander, Lieutenant

General John Abrams. General Abrams was a well-respected, soldier-focused leader who wanted to see how the medical infrastructure was progressing. The quality of the health care team that we had assembled was nothing short of superb. General Abrams made it known that he was extremely pleased with all the great work the unit had done. As a result of that late-night encounter, I believe we established the necessary rapport with the senior leadership team and their confidence, and as a direct result of that, we enjoyed their unwavering support throughout the entire mission. At the same time that we were providing support to our soldiers in the Balkans, the remainder of our nursing and health care team was back in Germany going through a Joint Commission survey. As a direct result of the preparation we had done prior to deployment and the Herculean efforts by my deputy and the Army reserve nurses and physicians brought in to fill the vacancies left by those deployed to Hungary, the hospital achieved extremely high results during the survey process. This was a truly remarkable accomplishment under the most challenging of circumstances.

In 1997, I was selected to attend a 1-year senior leadership course at the Army War College in Carlisle, PA. During the 1990s, only one ANC officer was sent to the war college per year. I was not the first person selected, but rather the second. The first officer selected had decided to retire within a year of the selection process and, therefore, could not attend the course. It was then that I was called and asked to attend. If the other officer had not retired, I would not have gone to the Army War College and, therefore, would never have been selected as chief of the Army Nurse Corps. Dad had said it—timing is everything. During my year at the Army War College, the Army changed its policy and opened up hospital command positions to all corps within the Army Medical Department, not just to the Medical Corps (physicians) as had been the policy previously. The first board convened in 1997 and selected the hospital commanders for 1999. Four nurses were selected to be included on this first list. I was fortunate enough to be one of those four.

Then, in the spring of 1998, I was called and notified that one of the commanders slated to command the Army Hospital at Ft. Jackson, SC, had been diverted to another assignment and I would be moved up a year early to serve in command. Therefore, in August 1998 I assumed command of Moncrieff Army Community Hospital and had the honor of being the first board-selected nonphysician to command an Army hospital. Once again, I was surrounded by unbelievable talent. There was consternation among some individuals about nonphysicians becoming CEOs of hospitals. Fortunately for me, the deputy commander for clinical services (the physician in charge of all the physicians) was an extremely talented, articulate, and objective professional. This officer put to rest any doubt and discontent very early on in my tenure. I can honestly say that my working relationship with this officer was as productive, pleasant, and rewarding as any relationship I had during my 30 years of military service. I also had the good fortune of having a director of nursing who was the total professional package: caring, funny, intelligent, experienced, visionary, and loved by her entire staff. She was a professional who cut to the point. During our first meeting, she said to me point-blank, "Well sir, you've been a director of nursing four times. Are you going to be the chief nurse here, or am I?" We quickly resolved that issue with my statement that I had plenty of work on my plate and did not intend to get involved with her responsibilities unless asked or needed. Needless to say, we are still very close friends today.

Probably the biggest surprise in my life occurred in February 2000. Our hospital was in the midst of a 4-day Joint Commission survey. I returned home late that evening and was having a glass of wine with my wife, Cheryl, when the doorbell rang. Cheryl answered the door and I heard her say, "Come in, sir." I immediately knew this had to be my boss, Major General Ray Barrett, but I couldn't figure out why he was visiting the house so late in the evening. He and his wife, Joan, had a bottle of champagne and he said, "Let's celebrate." My initial thought was that he mistakenly believed that the survey was over. But instead, he said, "Tomorrow they're going to announce your selection to brigadier general." This news took me so much by surprise that I was pretty much speechless. I had never considered myself a serious contender for the ANC chief position, and seriously never thought that I would see a male ANC chief during my professional career.

One of the first decisions (and certainly one of the most important of my term as ANC chief) I needed to make was selecting my deputy. The assistant chief of the ANC is the individual who runs the day-to-day operations of the corps and is responsible for ensuring that the needed communication and actions of the many members of staff and the clinical leadership throughout the ANC occur effectively and efficiently. I had made the decision that I wanted a deputy who had different skill sets than my own. I figured that would afford us the broadest base of knowledge in serving the approximately 3,400 active duty nurses, 25,009 civilian nurses, and some 8,000 reserve nurses. I selected Colonel Debbie Gustke, a well-known, talented, and experienced senior nurse who made the decision to forego command in order to assume the duties of assistant corps chief. It was by far the best decision I made during my tenure as chief of the Army Nurse Corps.

During our tenure as the leadership team for the Army Nurse Corps, we addressed some very significant issues. First, the United States became a nation at war in 2001. We were challenged daily by the requirement to provide nurses to support the war effort while, at the same time, providing adequate nursing personnel to support the health care mission here in the United States. In 2001, we deployed a total of 722 ANC officers. We deployed 1,001 officers in 2002 and 1,456 in 2003, and the number in 2004, when we left office, was projected to easily surpass the deployment number for 2003.

The critical national nursing shortage had a significant impact on our recruiting efforts, adding to our deployment challenges. In an attempt to increase our ability to recruit registered nurses into the Army, we increased our accession bonus from $5,000 to $10,000. We fought for and obtained $18 million for student loan repayment. We also increased the number of nursing schools with ROTC programs from 44 to 200, and increased the number of scholarships available for our Army Enlisted Commissioning Program from 55 to 85 per year. This latter program takes our talented enlisted soldiers and pays for them to go to nursing school. They then return to the Army as ANC commissioned officers.

We also approached the issue of nurse retention from a number of angles. We were able to increase the nurse anesthesia bonus for individuals who sign a two-year versus a one-year contract. We were able to maintain our monies for civilian graduate education during a time of extreme military fiscal cutbacks. We did, however, have to put an upper limit on the tuition that we could pay. Also at this time, we were confronted with a crippling hiring bureaucracy that required nearly four months of processing time to hire a new civilian nurse. This was troublesome since 50% of nurses in Army hospitals are civilians. We obtained a direct-hire authority that decreased that timeframe to 24 days and markedly improved our overall staffing strength of civilian nurses. We also focused on bolstering our investment in nursing research. In conjunction with the other Federal Nursing Service Chiefs (FNSCs), and with the unending support of U.S. Senator Daniel Inouye (D-HI), we were able to maintain the receipt of $6 million per year for tri-service (Army, Navy, and Air Force) nursing research. When I left office, our nurses were conducting over 90 studies. Also, in collaboration with the FNSCs, we began a perioperative clinical nurse specialist program and a doctoral (PhD) program in nursing at the Uniformed Services University of the Health Sciences in Bethesda, MD. Due to these and other efforts, our retention rate was the best it had been in many years, with only an 8.7% turnover rate in 2003.

Being the first male to serve as a chief of any of the service nurse corps is a very humbling honor. Many individuals have asked me, "Weren't we way overdue for a male chief of the corps?" I don't know that we were "overdue," but the time was certainly getting closer. We must remember that it was only in 2004 that we selected our first female physician general officer and our first female medical service corps general officer. The

Dental Corps has still not selected a female general officer. The fact that I was the one that ended up becoming the first male ANC chief is more a matter of timing than of talent. We have had great male talent for years in the ANC, and any number of senior male ANC officers who preceded me would have made outstanding corps chiefs. I was just lucky enough to be in the right place at the right time—more than once.

Some years back, the chief of the ANC adopted dual roles. Consequently, during my first two years as corps chief, I also served as the assistant surgeon general for force projection. In this role, I was responsible for the oversight of five directorates at the Office of the Surgeon General. These directorates included quality management, health care operations, Reserve affairs, health policy and services, and personnel. The responsibilities were great in this position and I was very thankful for the many quality professionals with whom I was once again surrounded. Of personal importance, during this time, I was housed in the Pentagon. The tragedy of 9/11 occurred on my watch. The pace of events, the activity, and the disruption at the Pentagon that resulted from that tragic day are things I'll never forget.

My final two years as corps chief found me assuming the role of commander of the Center for Health Promotion and Preventive Medicine. This elite organization of over 1,000 very specialized and talented professionals was responsible for all preventive medicine, environmental, and health promotion issues throughout the Army. This organization's broad scope encompassed such diversified issues as West Nile virus; pre- and postdeployment health surveys; mad-cow disease; environmental samples from areas around the world where our troops were deployed; training injuries throughout the Army; industrial hygiene and occupational health issues; ergonomically related injuries; dietary supplements; disease surveillance; laser and optical radiation safety; radio-frequency radiation; safe drinking water; anthrax vaccine; pregnancy and postpartum physical training programs; noise and hearing loss; and depleted uranium, to name just a few.

I closed out my military career on June 1, 2004. It was a career that spanned 32 years, involving 18 different assignments, two deployments, and the opportunity to experience a multitude of professional nursing experiences. Upon my retirement from the military, my wife and I took 6 months off and retreated to the woods and lakes of northern Wisconsin. During this retreat, in August 2004, I accepted a position as professor of clinical nursing at the University of Texas in Austin. I thought that life would now be settled, stable, and predictable. But then, in January 2005, I was proved wrong.

We had just returned from Christmas vacation in northern Minnesota when I received a phone call from Project Hope, a nongovernmental organization that has been engaged for the past 50 years in assisting needy or devastated communities in establishing a medical infrastructure and providing medical assistance and training. Project Hope invited me to lead the nursing portion of a health care team that was being sent to Indonesia to respond to the devastation caused by the tsunami on December 26, 2004. However, as a current employee of the University of Texas, I could not agree to a commitment to this project without university approval. The next day, I received a call from the university telling me that they approved my participation in this relief effort and wished me well. The following day I was on a plane to Hawaii to rendezvous with the U.S. Navy hospital ship, the USNS *Mercy*.

When our health care team arrived in Banda Aceh, Indonesia, we found a city of 400,000 people almost totally devastated. Some 150,000 people had perished in that area alone. The community's appreciation of the medical and nursing assistance we provided was far beyond what any of us had imagined. We became a part of their community, as they too became a part of ours. Together we worked long and hard at reestablishing health, order, and structure in their lives. It was, by far, one of the most rewarding experiences of my nursing career.

CONCLUSION

My career in Army nursing has afforded me a multitude of professional experiences in a variety of professional settings. Army nursing provides the type of opportunities that most nurses actively pursue throughout their professional career, and provides these opportunities in a proactive and extremely well structured professional development plan. The ANC has set the professional educational standard by establishing the bachelor's degree in nursing as the minimum entry-level requirement. This requirement has been in place since the mid-1970s. In addition, Army nursing has established formal 4-month clinical courses in critical care, emergency, psychiatric, perioperative, obstetrics/gynecology, and community health nursing. These courses provide outstanding preparation for our young nurses interested in any of the aforementioned specialties. All Army nurses are expected to obtain their master's degree no later than midway through their professional military career. The Army supports this endeavor by funding over 100 nurses per year to obtain graduate education. Additionally, the ANC funds four to six nurses to pursue doctoral education, after which graduates fill critical teaching and research positions throughout military health care facilities worldwide.

The opportunities for career advancement far surpass the opportunities usually experienced in civilian nursing. During my 32-year career in the ANC, I was promoted six times, each promotion resulting in a pay raise. In addition, I received annual pay raises and received longevity pay raises every two years. I truly believe that the clinical, teaching, and administrative opportunities I received far exceeded any expectations I could have had in any other professional nursing environment.

More importantly, I have been unbelievably fortunate to have worked with and for some of the most outstanding teachers, mentors, and leaders in nursing. It is to these individuals that I will be forever grateful. I have referred to but a few in this chapter. Many others had a significant influence on my clinical skills, my management style, and my leadership abilities. I will never be able to fully repay each of these individuals for the significant positive impact they have had on me, both personally and professionally. I only hope that by passing along some of the skills, wisdom, and experiences they shared with me to those just starting their nursing careers, I can keep their energy, their interest in advancing our profession, and their vision alive for some years to come.

REFERENCES

American Nurses Association. (1942, November). *Service of men nurses during war.* Washington, DC: Author.

Boivin, J. (2002). Men make their mark in military nursing. *Nursing Spectrum.* Retrieved October 21, 2005, from http://community.nursingspectrum.com/MagazineArticles/article.cfm?AID = 7906

Craig, L. N. (1956). Another goal achieved. *Nursing Outlook, 4*(3), 175–176.

Musser, H. R. (1941). Nurse or soldier? [Letter to the editor]. *American Journal of Nursing, 41,* 1449.

Proud to serve: The evolution of male Army Nurse Corps officers. (n.d.). Retrieved October 21, 2005, from http://history.amedd.army.mil/ANCWebsite/articles/malenurses.htm

Terriberry, W. S. (1908). The military nurse! A problem of demand and supply. *Journal of the Military Service Institution of the United States, 48,* 444–451.

PART II

Current Issues

Recently, a colleague and I were discussing our experiences as men in nursing. Over a cup of coffee, we shared personal anecdotes about being pressured by female colleagues to think, act, and behave as women do in order to function as nurses and integrate smoothly into our respective work settings and the profession. We both chuckled at the absurdity of it all, finding humor in our experiences as if they were somehow imbedded in the script of a television sitcom. But after the laughter, a tense and reflective silence followed. We both recognized the stress we felt as a result of these experiences, a stress that often remains hidden and unspoken.

If one is to believe the popular press and the psychological literature, men often have difficulty recognizing and articulating challenges stemming from personal relationships. We men nurses have relationships with ourselves, with our female nurse colleagues, and with the nursing profession. Gendered differences in those relationships have spurred many challenges. I believe these challenges are recognizable, at least among men. However, these challenges have rarely been discussed in the nursing literature. As a result, I don't believe it's just that "women don't get it" when it comes to the challenges men face as nurses; it's also that our female colleagues just aren't aware of those challenges. The following chapters aim to change this situation. The authors of the chapters in part II articulate some of the challenges for men in their intraprofessional nursing relationships. Such articulation is of vital importance. It is only after gendered challenges are brought to the discussion table that nursing can make strides in improving intraprofessional gendered relations.

—Chad E. O'Lynn

CHAPTER FIVE

The Effects of Gender on Communication and Workplace Relations

Christina G. Yoshimura and Sara E. Hayden

INTRODUCTION

If popular books, television shows, and news reports are to be believed, women and men are fundamentally different and those differences affect everything from how relationships are talked about to how friends and coworkers interact. But are the assumptions about male and female differences really true or do they simply reflect and perpetuate outdated stereotypes? The answer lies somewhere between these two options. Research suggests that there are real differences in men's and women's communication behaviors. However, that same research reveals that men and women are far more similar than they are different, and that there is often more variation within the sexes than between the sexes (Canary & Dindia, 1998; Lippa, 2002; Wood, 2005). Further complicating matters, differences in men's and women's communication patterns are rooted, at least in part, in gender, and gender is a social construct. As a result, as society changes so too do the gendered aspects of men's and women's communication (Canary & Dindia, 1998; Wood, 2005). The research that informs this chapter is based on current societal norms in the United States, and the conclusions offered here may not extend past these norms. Nonetheless, it is fair to say that in the contemporary United States, the differences between masculine and feminine communication patterns are both small *and* significant.

When people enter into a communication situation with differing assumptions, norms, and interpretations of communication behaviors, miscommunication often occurs. Miscommunication in the workplace can result in hurt feelings, tense relationships with coworkers and clients, stress, burnout, and work-related mistakes (Starkey, 2004; Tannen, 1994). When it comes to navigating gendered patterns of communication in the workplace, male nurses face a unique challenge. Unlike the situation in most professions, in nursing, women outnumber men by a significant margin (Spratley, Johnson, Sochalski, Fritz, & Spencer, 2001; Williams, 2004); moreover, as a care-based activity, nursing enacts stereotypically feminine behaviors and norms (Ekstrom, 1999). As a result, men in nursing likely encounter a work situation in which the predominant communication patterns among their peers are feminine.

This chapter begins with a discussion of the sex/gender distinction and a review of basic principles of communication. Next, information about typical patterns of masculine and feminine communication is addressed, and some of the implications of those patterns for male nurses are explored. Hopefully, this information will encourage readers to understand communication patterns as nonfixed and to recognize the value of developing flexibility in communication behaviors.

SEX/GENDER

Although often used interchangeably, sex and gender are two distinct, albeit related, concepts. Sex refers to the biological differences between male and female bodies—chromosomes, hormones, internal and external genitalia, and secondary sex characteristics. Gender, on the other hand, references the social and cultural assumptions, patterns, and behaviors that are associated with biological sex. For example, the fact that baby girls are typically wrapped in pink blankets and baby boys are typically wrapped in blue blankets reflects gender, not sex.

The pink and blue example is deceptively simple, however. Although it is unlikely that there is a biological basis for color choice, other issues are not so clear. For example, are the differences between women's and men's tendencies to engage in task-oriented behaviors the result of nature or of nurture? Although scholars continue to debate these questions, most agree that it is a mistake to insist on either/or answers (Bem, 1974; Lippa, 2002). Nature and nurture are profoundly intertwined. Even when there is a biological impulse or basis for behavior, that behavior is filtered through social processes and norms. For the purposes of this discussion, it is enough to recognize that socialization plays a significant role in the behaviors, attitudes, and assumptions of men and women. The study of gender, in turn, involves an examination of socialization processes and their implications.

Scholars seeking to understand and explain the process of gender acquisition draw on theoretical concepts from various academic disciplines including psychology, sociology, anthropology, philosophy, and communication studies. Although the specifics of the explanatory mechanisms differ, what the theories share in common is the understanding of gender as something that is *learned* and *reinforced* through interactions with others, including family members, friends, teachers, coworkers, and even strangers; *maintained* and/or *altered* through social institutions including schools, churches, businesses, and the media; and *internalized* and *performed* by individuals who respond to various factors including biological impulses, the psychological desire to fit in, personal goals and desires, and the messages they receive from others (Canary & Dindia, 1998; Lippa, 2002).

Consider the following example: Bob and Sue have a son, Thomas, whom they love very much. Like most parents, they offer guidance meant to encourage him to develop into a well-adjusted, responsible adult. As part of that guidance, from the time Thomas is very young Bob and Sue urge him to be tough in the face of pain or disappointment, reiterating a common cultural message, "Big boys don't cry." This message is repeated and reinforced by Thomas's playground friends, who tease him when he tears up after falling; by the movies and TV shows that Thomas enjoys, especially those featuring superheroes played by Vin Diesel and Arnold Schwarzenegger; and by his gym teacher, who urges him to keep pushing himself to run more laps even though Thomas has insisted that he is too tired to run any further. These and similar messages are repeated as Thomas grows, leading him to internalize the belief that real men are tough and don't show emotion. As a result, Thomas develops into a stoic man who courageously faces difficult situations without showing his fear, pain, or disappointment.

Importantly, however, this is not to say that Thomas and other men who have internalized the lesson "boys don't cry" will *never* respond to a situation emotionally. Whereas the differences between male and female bodies are relatively distinct, the differences between masculine and feminine behaviors are far murkier. Psychologists largely embraced the idea that masculinity and femininity were polar points on a single continuum until the early 1970s, when a pioneering researcher, Sandra Bem (1974), argued that masculinity and femininity are best understood as two separate dimensions. Bem's insight implies that individuals enact varying degrees of both masculinity and femininity. Bem developed a survey, the Bem Sex Role Inventory, through which the levels of a person's masculinity and femininity can be measured. She argued that a person who scores high on the masculinity scale and low on the femininity scale is likely to behave in predominantly masculine ways; a person who scores high on the femininity scale and low on the masculinity scale is likely to behave in predominantly feminine ways; and a person who scores high on both masculinity and femininity is likely to enact both masculine and feminine behaviors. These descriptions, however, reflect the extremes: People score at many different points on the masculinity and femininity scales.

Bem's insights ushered in a more sophisticated understanding of gender differences. Perhaps most importantly, Bem shows that gender attributes are complex and that gender behaviors are flexible. Whether an individual enacts feminine or masculine characteristics reflects multiple influences, including the demands of the situation, the expectations of the people with whom the individual is interacting, and the individual's skills, attitudes, and goals. Let's return to Thomas, the hypothetical example of a boy who has internalized the belief that real men don't express emotion in the face of disappointment. If Thomas chooses to pursue a career as a nurse, he may find himself involved in situations where patients have been emergently injured. Thomas's ability to prioritize physiological tasks rather than focusing on the patient's emotional state is an important skill in such instances, making him a valuable member of the health care team. In nonemergent situations, however, Thomas might find that it is useful to acknowledge and empathize with a patient's feelings of pain, fear, and discomfort. In these cases, Thomas will need to call on skills and behaviors more consistently linked to femininity. As has been described, Thomas's internalization of the lesson that men don't express emotion is particularly strong—in other words, he's one of those people who would probably score high on Bem's (1974) masculinity scale but low on the femininity scale. As such, he may find himself struggling to enact empathic behaviors. The good news, however, is that Thomas is not stuck. He can learn to recognize when certain behaviors are called for and to enact those behaviors even if they are not currently part of his usual behavioral repertoire. People are able to do this because differences in gendered behaviors are a matter of *degree* rather than *kind* (Wood & Dindia, 1998). Both men and women express emotion, disclose intimate information, engage in competition, and concern themselves with status. It is only the degree to which men and women are socialized to do each of these things that differs.

In sum, gender is best understood as a multidimensional social construct, learned through interaction with others, internalized by individuals, and expressed through our behaviors, actions, and attitudes. Gender identities are composed of both masculine and feminine characteristics. Expressions of those characteristics reflect people's responses to situations and to other people, and people's skills, desires, and goals. One of the primary ways gender is enacted is through communication.

COMMUNICATION

In spite of what authors like Emily Post might suggest, there are no right or wrong communication behaviors. Rather, beliefs about what kinds of communication fall in line with good manners reflect norms learned and enacted in families, communities, peer groups, and workplaces. A useful way to understand this is through the concept of a speech community (Labov, 1972). A speech community exists when people share goals for communication behavior, norms for achieving those goals, and interpretations of communication events. For example, a nurse working in a pediatrician's office likely finds himself in a speech community in which one of the initial goals of communication is to comfort and relax both the young patients and their parents. The norms for achieving this goal might include engaging in small talk about favorite television shows, toys, or daily activities. If the exchange goes well, these communication behaviors are interpreted as signs of compassion, professionalism, and concern with getting the job done right; the nurse is then in a position to turn to more task-oriented behaviors. In contrast, a nurse in a busy emergency room likely finds himself in an entirely different sort of speech community. Especially in emergency situations, the initial goals of communication will be to transmit information quickly and accurately. The norms for achieving these goals might include asking specific questions in order to elicit information about the patient's health; little time or effort will be spent on small talk until the crisis has abated. If the exchange goes well, once again the patient will interpret the nurse's communication as a sign of compassion, professionalism, and concern with getting the job done correctly.

Although the nurses in both situations hope to achieve the same results—to express compassion, professionalism, and concern for their patients—they do so in different ways. Further, the nurses' goals might not be met. In fact, in either scenario, miscommunication might very well occur. One of the main causes of miscommunication is that people do not share the same rules of communication; they are not members of the same speech communities. As professionals in a medical setting, nurses participate in a medical speech community on a regular basis; clients do not. Even though clients likely share the same goals as nurses—to maintain, improve, and/or protect their own health—they do not necessarily share the rules of communication that the nurse has come to understand as appropriate for a medical setting. As a result, the parent with whom a nurse engages in small talk might misinterpret that behavior as an effort to establish an ongoing friendship or personal relationship. Similarly, the patient in the emergency room might interpret a nurse's efficiency and focus on psychomotor tasks as a sign of a lack of compassion or concern.

The potential for miscommunication is increased as a result of the multiple speech communities in which participants exist. Thus far the focus of this chapter has been on the speech communities specific to various medical settings. However, speech communities are also formed as a result of other factors, including geographic location, ethnicity, and most important for our purposes here, gender.

Boys and Girls in Communication

From the moment a baby is wrapped in those pink or blue blankets at birth, the child receives messages about gender. Those messages simultaneously identify the gender the child is to enact and specify the particular behaviors that are appropriate for that gender. The example of Thomas alluded to one of the messages boys receive about masculinity—that boys should be tough in the face of pain. In addition to this, boys are also expected to be active and energetic. They are often encouraged to play in competitive sports and to excel in school and in other intellectual pursuits. Girls, on the other hand, are taught that they should be pleasant, kind, friendly, and sweet. They are not to be too loud or aggressive. In school they often receive more praise for being neat and orderly than for being smart. As Wood (2005) points out, girls and boys often play in same-sex groups, and the messages about masculinity and femininity they receive from parents, peers, and social institutions are reinforced through the games they play in those groups. Girls, for example, will often play games that promote nurturing and affiliative behaviors such as playing house or school or engaging in arts and crafts. These games, in conjunction with the messages girls receive about femininity, lead to the development of a girls' speech community with at least these four rules:

1. Use communication to create and maintain relationships. The process of communication, not its content, is the heart of relationships.
2. Use communication to establish egalitarian relations with others. Don't outdo, criticize, or put others down. If you have to criticize, be gentle.
3. Use communication to include others—bring them into conversations, respond to their ideas.

4. Use communication to show sensitivity to others and relationships. (Wood, 2005, p. 118)

Boys, on the other hand, are more likely to structure their play around
more competitive, aggressive settings, including sports or video games.
In combination with the messages they receive about masculinity, boys'
games lead to the development of a speech community with these rules:

1. Use communication to assert your ideas, opinions, and identity.
2. Use talk to achieve something, such as solving problems or
   developing strategies.
3. Use communication to attract and maintain others' attention.
4. Use communication to compete for the "talk stage." Make yourself stand out; take attention away from others and get others to
   pay attention to you. (Wood, 2005, p. 117)

While of course children will adopt these rules to varying degrees depending on the other messages and influences they receive, in broad terms,
these rules shape the patterns of communication behavior children learn
when they are young. Importantly, these rules continue to shape communication behaviors as children grow and develop.

Men and Women in Communication

By adulthood, the cumulative effect of socialization in gendered speech
communities can result in some significant differences in communication
behaviors. Gray (1992) suggests that differences between the communication preferences and behaviors of men and women are so vast that men
may as well be from Mars and women may as well be from Venus. In
contrast, Dindia argues that the differences in communication between
men and women are less dichotomous and drastic, so that it may seem
that men are from North Dakota and women are from South Dakota
(Wood & Dindia, 1998).

The perspective advocated in this chapter is that men and women
are overwhelmingly communicating in nearly identical ways. In support
of this perspective, Mulac (1998) found over the course of several studies
that the average person could not actually discern whether a speaking
sample was created by a man or a woman, indicating that the differences
cannot possibly be as prevalent and obvious as several popular authors
propose. However, even though respondents in Mulac's studies couldn't
consciously tell whether language was created by a man or a woman,
there were nonetheless slight differences in how they judged the language
sample. Specifically, the language produced by women was consistently

rated as being of a higher status and more pleasant, and the language produced by men was consistently rated as being more dynamic and strong. To be consistently rated in this way, the communication of men and women must have small differences that, nonetheless, significantly impact how that communication is perceived.

Communication and the Nursing Profession

Nursing is one of the few remaining professions in the United States that is female dominated, and as such, the conventions for communication remain strongly influenced by female speech communities. Men in nursing may initially be struck by the impact these speech communities can have on communication among nurses. It's important to remember that, regardless of conventions for communication, every instance of communication imparts both a content and a relational message (Watzlawick, Beavin, & Jackson, 1967). Consider, for example, the simple question, "How are you today?" The content level of communication refers to the denotative meaning, or the dictionary definitions of the words used. The relational level of the message refers to everything but the content that the message conveys. The context in which the words are spoken, the tone of voice or gestures that accompany the words, and even the specific phrasing choices ("How are y'all?" versus "How's it going?" versus "How are you today?") communicate the feelings of the communicators in the interaction, and the relationship between the communicators. So, for example, when people pass colleagues in the hall they might say, "How's it going?" using the question as a quick greeting to indicate familiarity and friendship. However, if this question is posed by a nurse to a patient who is recovering from heart surgery, the meaning will be quite different, reinforcing the relationship between the nurse as professional caretaker and the patient as the care-receiver, a difference that will be reflected in the form the question takes ("How are you today?" rather than "How's it going?"), the setting, tone of voice, and subsequent interactions. Finally, the same question posed by a loved one would mean something different yet again. This time, the question likely reflects feelings of personal concern and the desire for an intimate connection. *Relationship messages and content messages are sent by both men and women in every interaction.* However, the difference in gendered speech communities emerges when we look at the relative focus placed on these two levels of messages.

Following from the rules first established in girlhood, female speech communities emphasize more of the relational nature of communication, using verbal and nonverbal messages together to communicate information about equality, support, and relational status. Tannen (1994) refers to this as "rapport talk"—communication that is focused on establishing, evaluating, and maintaining affiliation with a partner in conversation. Male speech communities socialize members to emphasize more of the content level of communication, to focus on instrumental goals and command. Tannen calls this "rapport talk"—communication focused on accomplishing tasks. As nursing is a profession dominated by women, it seems likely that nurses frequently engage in rapport talk among themselves. This might include sharing information about one another's families, including relationships with romantic partners, children, and aging parents. Similarly, nurses might regularly discuss relatively insignificant events, including where they purchased the fabric they plan to use for their child's Halloween costume or the movie they would like to see over the weekend. For the women involved, these conversations do more than fill time. They establish relationships of mutual support and respect that serve as the basis for their interactions in the workplace. If the small number of male nurses in the predominantly female nursing group does not conform to the rapport talk emphasis in the workplace, the nurses will still be able to function in their duties without too much difficulty. However, the male nurses are likely to wonder when the female nurses will get to the point, and the female nurses may be concerned that the male nurses are withdrawn or unfriendly.

Giving and receiving praise is another issue that is affected by the differences between report and rapport talk. The norms of feminine communication lead women to both give and expect praise on a regular basis. For feminine communicators, praise often functions to let another person know that his efforts are appreciated and noticed; as a result, it becomes a matter of routine. The norms of masculine communication, with an emphasis on accomplishing goals and getting things done, lead to less frequent use of praise. Typically when men give praise they do so in response to what they perceive to be particularly well-done tasks or significant accomplishments. The issue of giving praise might lead to tension between men and women in the workplace. If a nursing context is marked by feminine norms, including the regular doling out of praise and appreciation, the male nurse who receives this praise may begin to think that his work is better than average. Conversely, because he is not in the habit of giving out praise for ordinary efforts, the women he works with might feel he does not recognize or appreciate their efforts, and they might perceive him as particularly cold or arrogant.

These are just two examples of possible miscommunications in the workplace that can result from the differences between masculine and feminine communication norms.

At this point, it is important to point out that neither the masculine nor the feminine style is superior to the other. People who use either style are equally committed to achieving excellence in the workplace and cordial relations with coworkers. They simply go about these tasks in different ways. Moreover, although neither style is inherently better than the other, it is true that depending on the situation, one style might be more useful or appropriate than the other. It was suggested above that a nurse working in an emergency situation will seek to transmit information quickly and accurately. He will give priority to direct questioning in order to learn specific information; and he will give less priority to friendly small talk. These communication behaviors largely reflect a masculine communication style. Conversely, it was also suggested that an important goal for a nurse working in a pediatrician's office would be to relax the young patients and their parents. A nurse in this situation is likely to engage in small talk about inconsequential topics, showing direct interest in and concern for the people with whom he is working. These communication behaviors largely reflect a feminine communication style.

Communication Accommodation Theory (CAT) indicates that adjusting one's speech and mannerisms to match the communication patterns of others indicates affiliation and liking (Street & Giles, 1982). Thus, both for the sake of good workplace interactions between colleagues and to meet the varied goals in medical settings, it is useful to develop flexibility in communication behaviors. Some convergence of speech styles will be likely to yield a workplace with mutual respect among coworkers and excellence in nursing care. Both men and women should be aware of, and responsive to, the communication patterns of both male and female speech communities.

While both masculine and feminine communication patterns can be useful in the nursing profession, there are two areas of communication where people who utilize a primarily masculine style of communication might be at a disadvantage—nonverbal communication behaviors and the expression of emotion. Because these communication forms are particularly important for nurses (Eckstrom, 1999; McCabe, 2004), they deserve particular attention here.

Nonverbal Behavior

Nonverbal behaviors are commonly considered to be all the messages communicated through nonlinguistic means. Tone of voice, speaking rate, and use of pauses are all forms of nonverbal communication, just like those that more commonly come to mind, such as body movement, touch, eye contact, and spatial proximity. In the film *In and Out* (Rudin & Rudnick, 1997), for example, Kevin Kline's character listens to an audio tape describing the vocal tone, dress, and movements that "real men" must use. Perhaps no other area of communication is as strongly policed by our society, in the desire that men and women conform to set roles. As such, nonverbal communication is one area of communication that the average person attends to very closely, and an area in which people *can* distinguish between male and female behaviors (Briton & Hall, 1995).

However, in the female-dominant profession of nursing, male nurses find themselves perplexed to discover that many of the nonverbal attributes that they have been encouraged to display throughout their lives by peers, the media, and other people are not those that are most congruous to the historical nurturing roles of nursing. For instance, in comparison to women, men exhibit limited variation in inflection while speaking, engage in more frequent interruptions, limit eye contact with others, maintain more personal space, and use touch to direct others rather than to indicate affection, support, or comfort (Wood, 2005). Overall, research shows that women exhibit more frequent and varied nonverbal behaviors and greater skill at decoding the nonverbal behaviors of others than do men (Noller, 1986). This certainly makes sense considering the communication rules that girls learn. Again, the norms of femininity encourage girls to use communication to create and maintain relationships and to show sensitivity to others. Attending to nonverbal messages plays a large part in these efforts.

Several researchers have found that patients appreciated nurses and other health care providers being friendly and attentive, especially by using nonverbal behaviors to show their commitment to and liking of the patient (Conlee, Olvera, & Vagim, 1993; McCabe, 2004). Women's greater use of and experience working with nonverbal behaviors puts them at an advantage in creating this form of patient satisfaction within the nurse-patient relationship, but men can quite easily expand their nonverbal communication repertoire with training (Keeley-Dyreson, Burgoon, & Bailey, 1991; Rosenthal & DePaulo, 1979) and with mindfulness of behaviors exhibited at work. Moving entirely toward a feminine style of nonverbal communication is not necessary, but taking into account behaviors intended to show liking and affiliation (termed "immediacy behaviors") could prove useful in communicating attention and friendliness to patients.

Common immediacy behaviors that may be used successfully by male nurses include reducing physical distance to the space necessary to conduct a conversation that cannot be heard more than a few feet away, maintaining eye contact while the patient is speaking, facing the patient as much as possible during interactions, and leaning slightly toward patients while speaking with them (Andersen, 1985; Berger & Diggs, 2002). Although nurses are understandably pressed for time, one nonverbal behavior that communicates a great deal of care and concern is willingness to spend time with patients and to indicate to patients that they are worth the time being spent on them. When it is not possible to communicate this nonverbally by remaining with the patient for a long span of time, apologizing for being rushed or otherwise communicating that the patient is valued may result in a sense of the nurse's care for the patient similar to that created by actual time spent by the bedside. Of course, these suggestions are guidelines that should be adjusted with careful consideration to patients' reactions to these nonverbal behaviors. Due to cultural differences, personal preferences, or any number of other factors, some patients may prefer an increased distance or feel uncomfortable with sustained eye contact. A careful focus on the nonverbal communication of the patient should guide the nurse's own communicative behaviors.

Expression of Emotion

Nurse educators have consistently emphasized to new nurses the need to show compassion to their patients (e.g., Forsyth, 1980; Holden, 1990). However, researchers have begun to suggest that expressions of understanding are not sufficient for nurse-patient interaction, but that *emotional empathy*, or emotional engagement of the nurse with the patient, is preferable (Morse, Bottorff, Anderson, O'Brien, & Solbert, 1992). This type of communication not only requires nurses to understand the patient's experience but also requires that they put themselves in the patient's place and identify with the suffering. Nurses can then reflect that emotion back to the patient, which results in satisfaction with the interaction on the part of the patient (McCabe, 2004). Morse et al. (1992) actually note that such emotional expression not only benefits the patient but may also reward the caregiver, as open expression may limit occupational burnout. Nurses' mental health is not achieved only through expression of emotion to patients but also through emotional expressions of social support between nursing coworkers. Success as a nurse may depend on the ability to give and receive emotional support (Jenkins & Elliott, 2004); in fact, most nurses report that they would seek the help of another nurse with a problem rather than seek managerial or outside assistance (Dallender, Nolan, Soares, Thomsen, & Arnetz, 1999).

There are many early socialization lessons through which boys may learn to become uncomfortable showing or responding to expressions of pain or similar emotions. In fact, some scholars even believe that men are evolutionarily programmed not to show much emotion, since controlling emotions such as fear may have been helpful to our male ancestors (see Buck, 1984). Whether the difference in emotional expression arises due to evolutionary reasons or due to socialization in different speech communities, the fact that most men tend to be less emotionally responsive and expressive than women is a salient issue in the nursing profession. Female coworkers and patients may feel unsupported and dismissed by a nurse who displays an orientation toward accomplishing instrumental tasks rather than establishing affiliation or tending to traditional ideas of nurturing. Yet, as is the case with nonverbal expressivity, men certainly have the capacity to express and interpret emotional communication messages that will yield success in the nursing profession. The key to utilizing these skills in a nursing context rests in adapting to the communication norms of nursing, rather than relying exclusively on the gendered messages many men have received throughout their lives regarding emotional behavior.

As nurses work to refine the emotional communication skills necessary to their profession, they may find it useful to engage in perspective-taking with coworkers and patients. This process involves describing the emotional messages received from a patient or coworker, then asking for ways to interpret these messages. For instance, Thomas may see a patient gazing at flowers that have been delivered to her while tears are streaming down her face. He could say, "I see that you're crying; what are you feeling right now?" Seeking feedback will help nurses learn to recognize nuances in a variety of emotional expressions, and questions like the one Thomas asked also show an interest in the emotional experiences of others. Often it is the interest, not just the accuracy, that can help make people feel valued and cared for.

SOURCES OF TENSION IN NURSING

There are several points at which gender norms and communication norms may intersect in the nursing profession, creating challenges for the nurses who must navigate them. These are identified here not to justify their existence, nor necessarily to suggest definitive solutions. However, it is useful to identify some of these sources of tension in order to open the door for nurses to confront their fears, concerns, and tensions together.

One potential source of friction or surprise for men in nursing may be the ambivalence female nurses are likely to communicate regarding the increasing proportion of male nurses in the workforce. Women may feel an interruption in the camaraderie of an all-girls' network, or feel uncomfortable about communication events such as bachelorette parties or baby showers, which have traditionally linked only the female coworkers in the workplace. Even more importantly, women may feel that due to the typically male upper administration in health care settings, men arriving in the nursing field will be able to procure the more preferred or lucrative positions rather than women who have more seniority or experience

(Williams, 2004). Patriarchal control and sexual harassment are common occurrences in many workplaces. Women may fear that bringing male nurses into the field means they will experience these communication behaviors from coworkers. (Although sexual harassment tends to be perpetuated predominantly by men in the workplace, it is important to note that it is behavior that women can and sometimes do utilize as well [Wood, 2005]. Sexual harassment should be understood as an exercise of power and intimidation and thus may occur with or without a male influence in the workplace. It is the *anticipation* of sexual harassment and control that may increase with the growing percentage of men in the field of nursing, not necessarily the *occurrence*.)

It is not necessarily the case that women will resist the increasing entrance of men into the nursing profession, however. In fact, many women may openly welcome more men into nursing. The higher status men still hold in U.S. society may be used as a way to bring more prestige to the nursing profession when male nurses are hired. Or women may enjoy enacting a nurturing role toward male nurses, due to their minority status in the nursing profession (Clair, 1994). Used to being in the minority in many workplace situations, women may feel pride at the opportunity to be in the majority among nurses and to coach male nurses who enter the profession. The reception that male nurses receive in nursing will have much to do with the communication culture that has been established in the department that they enter, the number of male nurses already on staff, and the prior experiences of the female nurses in the department in communicating with other men in the workplace situation.

Men may also anticipate resistance from society at large regarding their entry into the female-dominated nursing profession. Messages that men who enter traditionally female fields must be homosexual, wimpy, or desperate (Williams, 2004) mean that male nurses may suffer in regard to self-esteem and acceptance, particularly from other men. They may feel the need to communicate hypermasculine identities, yet at the same time, these identities can create another set of difficulties. Since gendered norms for behavior are so strongly socialized, a man who chooses to pursue a career in a field traditionally dominated by women may be perceived as having unscrupulous motives, such as the intent to abuse or manipulate. Male nurses must work carefully to ensure that their behavior and interaction patterns express compassion, equality, and sexual neutrality, in order to avoid being accused of impropriety, especially in intimate situations with women and children (Williams, 2004). Thus, neither feminine/neutral behavior nor hypermasculinity will communicate an identity that will satisfy all the groups that are potentially concerned about the role of men in nursing.

Finally, male nurses must navigate a complicated hierarchy in the workplace regarding their use of power and control. Although practices

typically associated with femininity are prevalent within the nursing profession, more masculine communication traits still hold sway in business overall. Administrators and managers in health care settings have
expectations and job responsibilities, arising from mainstream business
and financial concerns, that are seemingly different from the patient-care
emphasis of nurses on the front lines. Expressions of confidence, competitiveness, and independence are likely to be exhibited and sought by
members of health care organizations who occupy the more bureaucratic
levels of the organizational hierarchy. Nurses who have been socialized in
the male speech communities that are the basis of most professional settings (Wood, 2005) may find that they are better suited than their female
counterparts to using communication that is valued by administrators
and managers.

Yet, this competency in communicating with superiors may result
in resentment or confusion among female coworkers. The recognition
and advancement of male nurses adept at communicating with the upper
administration may be a source of contention among female nurses; especially those who find themselves equally technically competent or who
have similar seniority within the organization, yet find themselves unable
to engage in the same communication process with the administration
or to receive the same outcomes. Of course, one useful response to this
situation could be for female nurses to learn the norms of a masculine
communication style. This is one area where male nurses may serve as
mentors to their female colleagues. At the same time, both male and female nurses must find a way to communicate with coworkers in ways
that do not emphasize status or power. Both male and female nurses will
want to engage in considerable flexibility in their communication, in order to shift patterns when speaking with administrators/supervisors and
speaking with coworkers.

Finally, this flexibility must also come into play on yet another level
of the health care hierarchy: communication between nurse and patient.
Specifically, Hewison (1995) found that nurses tend to use four strategies
to achieve power over the patients for whom they are responsible:

1. *Overt communication*—confident, direct communication to tell
   the patient what is expected (e.g., "You need to take a walk
   down the hallway now.")
2. *Persuasion*—indirect communication used to gain patient compliance through questioning and repetition (e.g., "Are you sure
   you don't feel like a walk? Maybe you'd like to walk down the
   hall for just a few minutes?")
3. *Controlling the agenda*—references to patterns and routines to
   direct patient behavior (e.g., "After breakfast, all the patients
   take a walk down the hallway for a little exercise.")

4. *Terms of endearment*—communicating to patients in informal, endearing terms to ingratiate the patient to the nurse (e.g., "Now, dear, let's just get you up for a little walk now, hmm?")

Overt communication reflects the power strategies typically utilized in masculine speech communities, yet the other three strategies utilize qualities typically associated with feminine speech communities (such as emphasizing equality and cooperation over competition). Behavioral flexibility between typical feminine and masculine styles will be a practical skill in motivating patients. Such flexibility may also prove useful in negotiating the communication of power and control throughout the healthcare hierarchy, from patients to coworkers to doctors and administrators within the organization.

CONCLUSION

This chapter has reviewed the differences between sex and gender, discussed some of the ways gender is acquired, and investigated the implications of gender for communication patterns as they relate to workplace interaction. Although it has been argued here that men's and women's communication behaviors are more similar than different, small differences do exist between women's and men's communication styles. More so than women's, men's communication is likely to be task oriented and instrumental. The primary goal of communication is to get something done. More so than men's, women's communication is affiliative and relationship oriented. The primary goal of communication is to establish connections with others.

As nursing is a female-dominated profession, the norms of communication in nursing reflect women's speech communities. As more and more men enter the nursing profession, however, both male and female nurses will benefit from understanding how gender is reflected in nurses' communication norms and from developing flexibility in their communication behaviors. Not only will increased understanding and flexibility promote positive working relationships between coworkers but it will lead to better nursing care. The tasks, responsibilities, and duties of nurses are vast. In the course of a single day, a nurse may be asked to comfort a person whose family member has died; to distract a child who is afraid of receiving an injection; to accurately impart complex information about a patient's new drug regimen; to negotiate a schedule conflict with a coworker; and/or to act quickly and efficiently in the face of another's serious injury. No single set of communication behaviors is appropriate in all of these situations; rather, in order to be able to meet these varied demands, nurses must posses a wide array of communication skills that can be found in both masculine and feminine speech communities. This chapter provides a starting point for developing those skills.

REFERENCES

Andersen, P. A. (1985). Nonverbal immediacy in interpersonal communication. In A. W. Siegman & S. Feldsteisn (Eds.), *Multicultural integrations of nonverbal behavior* (pp. 1–36). Hillsdale, NJ: Erlbaum.
Bem, S. L. (1974). The measurement of psychological androgyny. *Journal of Consulting and Clinical Psychology, 42,* 155–162.
Berger, B. & Diggs, A. M. (2002). Immediacy—Part 2: Nonverbal communication. *US Pharmacist, 25*(8). Retrieved April 25, 2006 from http://www.uspharmacist.com/oldformat.asp?url=newlook/files/phar/aug00rel.htm
Briton, N. J., & Hall, J. A. (1995). Beliefs about female and male nonverbal communication. *Sex Roles, 32,* 79–90.
Buck, R. (1984). *The communication of emotion.* New York: Guilford Press.
Canary, D. J., & Dindia, K. (1998). *Sex differences and similarities in communication: Critical essays and empirical investigations of sex and gender in interaction.* Mahwah, NJ: Lawrence Erlbaum.
Clair, R. P. (1994). Resistance and oppression as a self-contained opposite: An organizational communication analysis of one man's story of sexual harassment. *Western Journal of Communication, 58,* 235–262.
Conlee, C. J., Olvera, J., & Vagim, N. N. (1993). The relationships among physician nonverbal immediacy and measures of patient satisfaction with physician care. *Communication Reports, 6,* 25–34.
Dallender, J., Nolan, P., Soares, J., Thomsen, S., & Arnetz, B. (1999). A comparative study of the perceptions of British mental health nurses and psychiatrists of their work environment. *Journal of Advanced Nursing, 29,* 36–43.
Eckstrom, D. N. (1999). Gender and perceived nurse caring in nurse-patient dyads. *Journal of Advanced Nursing, 29,* 1393–1401.
Forsyth, G. L. (1980). Analysis of the concept of empathy: Illustration of one approach. *Advances in Nursing Science, 2,* 33–42.
Gray, J. (1992). *Men are from Mars, women are from Venus: A practical guide for improving communication and getting what you want in your relationships.* New York: HarperCollins.
Hewison, A. (1995). Nurses' power in interaction with patients. *Journal of Advanced Nursing, 21,* 75–82.
Holden, R. J. (1990). Empathy: The art of emotional knowing in holistic nursing care. *Holistic Nursing Practice, 5,* 70–79.
Jenkins, R. & Elliott, P. (2004). Stressors, burnout and social support: Nurses in acute mental health settings. *Journal of Advanced Nursing, 48,* 622–631.
Keeley-Dyreson, M., Burgoon, J. K., & Bailey, W. (1991). The effects of stress and gender on nonverbal decoding accuracy in kinesic and vocalic channels. *Human Communication Research, 17,* 584–605.
Labov, W. (1972). *Sociolinguistic patterns.* Philadelphia: University of Pennsylvania Press.
Lippa, R. A. (2002). *Gender, nature, and nurture.* Mahwah, NJ: Lawrence Erlbaum.
McCabe, C. (2004). Nurse-patient communication: An exploration of patients' experiences. *Journal of Clinical Nursing, 13,* 41–49.

Morse, J. M., Bottorff, J., Anderson, G., O'Brien, B., & Solbert, S. (1992). Beyond empathy: Expanding expressions of caring. *Journal of Advanced Nursing, 17,* 809–821.

Mulac, A. (1998). The gender-linked language effect. Do language differences really make a difference? In D. Canary & K. Dindia (Eds.), *Sex differences and similarities in communication* (pp. 127–153). Mahwah, NJ: Erlbaum.

Noller, P. (1986). Sex differences in nonverbal communication: Advantage lost or supremacy regained? *Australian Journal of Psychology, 38,* 23–32.

Rosenthal, R. & DePaulo, B. M. (1979). Sex differences in accommodation in nonverbal communication. In R. Rosenthal (Ed.), *Skill in nonverbal communication: Individual differences* (pp. 68–103). Cambridge, MA: Oelgeschlager, Gunn, & Hain.

Rudin, S. (Producer) & Rudnick, P. (Writer). (1997). *In and out* [Motion picture]. United States: Paramount Pictures.

Spratley, E., Johnson, A., Sochalski, J., Fritz, M., & Spencer, W. (2001). *The registered nurse population March 2000: Findings from the national sample survey of registered nurses.* Washington, DC: U.S. Department of Health and Human Services, Bureau of Health Professions, Division of Nursing.

Starkey, S. M. (2004). *Women and men tending together: Gender and communication factors for nurses.* Unpublished professional paper, University of Montana, Missoula.

Street, R. L., Jr., & Giles, H. (1982). Speech accommodation theory: A social cognitive approach to language and speech behavior. In M. Roloff & C. Berger (Eds.), *Social cognition and communication* (pp. 193–226). Beverly Hills, CA: Sage.

Tannen, D. (1994). *Talking from 9 to 5: How women's and men's conversational styles affect who gets heard, who gets credit, and what gets done at work.* New York: William Morrow.

Watzlawick, P., Beavin, J., & Jackson, D. D. (1967). *Pragmatics of human communication.* New York: W. W. Norton.

Williams, C. L. (2004). The glass escalator: Hidden advantages for men in the "female" professions. In M. S. Kimmel & M. A. Messner (Eds.), *Men's lives* (6th ed., pp. 227–240). Boston: Allyn and Bacon.

Wood, J. T. (2005). *Gendered lives: Communication, gender and culture* (6th ed.). Belmont, CA: Wadsworth.

Wood, J. T., & Dindia, K. (1998). What's the difference? A dialogue about differences and similarities between women and men. In D. J. Canary and K. Dindia (Eds.), *Sex differences and similarities in communication: Critical investigations of sex and gender in interaction* (pp. 19–40). Mahwah, NJ: Lawrence Erlbaum.

CHAPTER SIX

Men, Caring, and Touch

Chad E. O'Lynn

INTRODUCTION

Perhaps no concept in nursing has been more studied yet remains more elusive than caring, despite the centrality nursing has placed on the concept (Morse, Bottorff, Neander, & Solberg, 1991; Morse, Solberg, Neander, Bottorff, & Johnson, 1990). Authors frequently cite Leininger, who for decades has boldly declared that caring is the essence of nursing, and who explains that not only does caring unify the profession with its dominant focus, but that caring also constitutes the heart and soul of nursing (Leininger, 1991). During her education as a nurse in the early 1940s, Leininger notes that she was instructed to give complete and comprehensive care to her clients, but was never taught "specific concepts about human care or caring. Caring was a taken-for-granted expectation ... [whose] very nature remained obscure" (p. 9). Leininger went on to develop the theory of Culture Care Diversity and Universality, and with colleagues and followers, has conducted numerous studies that describe similar and differing caring beliefs and actions among cultures. Likewise, numerous researchers and scholars have studied nurses and have proposed theories explaining how nurses care for clients. Yet, despite all this activity attempting to understand and explain caring, little research has been completed in the area of examining how male nurses, as men, care for and care about others.

In chapter 5 of this book, Yoshimura and Hayden describe the differences in communication patterns between men and women. The fact that there are differences should be of no surprise to most individuals, based on the number of books devoted to communication issues in male-female relationships. It is unclear, then, why little attention is given to masculine styles of care, particularly if caring *actions* communicate caring *feelings*. The communication styles associated with men are no better and no worse than the communication styles associated with women; however, some styles are more effective in certain contexts than others. Would the caring styles associated with men be more effective in certain contexts rather than others? If so, what are those styles and contexts? This chapter will first review the complexity of care as a concept and then summarize briefly what is known about men and caring. The chapter will then focus on touch, and the ways in which this behavior, described as central to caring, is problematic for many male nurses in today's society.

THE COMPLEXITY OF CARING

Nearly every author who discusses caring notes its complexity and its ability to defy definition. To add to the complexity, there are various uses of the term "care." Care is used in multiple ways as a verb, as in to care for or to care about an individual or object, the former being more instrumental in nature but the latter being more affective in nature. Care is also used in multiple ways as a noun, to mean an affect or trait or the collection of actions and behaviors that communicate caring. Clearly, the term is as complex as other terms that often have an assumed understanding, such as "love" or "happiness," terms that in reality are highly individualized in meaning, manifestations, and difficulty of measurement.

Within the nursing literature, two important meta-analyses have attempted to provide some semblance of clarity. The first was conducted by a team of nurse scholars headed by Janice Morse (Morse et al., 1990, 1991). In examining 35 nurse authors who had explicitly or implicitly defined caring and its related concepts, Morse et al. note that caring has five perspectives with two associated outcomes of caring. There are theoretical links among these perspectives. The perspectives include caring as a human trait, affect, moral imperative, interpersonal interaction, and therapeutic intervention. The two outcomes of caring are the client's subjective experience and the client's physical response to caring.

The first perspective, that caring is a human trait, implies that caring is innate and essential to human existence (Morse et al., 1990, 1991). As a trait, caring becomes a motivator of actions and behaviors indicative of caring. Authors report that this trait is not uniform and is highly influenced by sociocultural variables and personal experience. Caring as a trait has been analyzed as a phenomenon between individuals and among groups. The nursing theorists most associated with this perspective include Leininger, Ray, Roach, and Griffin. The second perspective, that caring is an affect, describes caring as a feeling of emotional involvement and empathy with others. Authors have suggested that this perspective also motivates actions and behaviors, and that in doing so, it strives toward mutual goals of self-actualization. Caring as affect predisposes an individual to vulnerability and altruism. In addition, environmental and relational barriers can prevent the display of this affectual nature of caring. The theorists describing this perspective include Forrest, Gendron, McFarlane, and Fanslow.

Caring as a moral imperative is a third perspective of caring (Morse et al., 1990, 1991). In this perspective, caring is described as a fundamental value, an ideal that can never quite be attained, yet one that forms a foundation for nursing action. Scholars such as Watson and Gadow highlight this perspective and suggest that care strives to maintain the dignity or integrity of clients. In contrast, other authors, such as Horner, Knowlden, Weiss, and Benner and Wrubel, suggest that the interpersonal relationships between nurses and clients not only display caring but are, in actuality, definitions of caring. Still others, such as Orem, Gaut, and Brown, present the fifth perspective, caring as therapeutic intervention. Rather than defining caring, these authors focus on behaviors and actions that communicate care. These actions may be "specific, such as attentive listening, patient teaching, patient advocacy, touch…or caring may include all nursing actions…that enable or assist patients" (Morse et al., 1990, p. 6). Beyond these perspectives, Morse et al. note that a number of researchers have examined caring not from the perspective of the nurse but instead in terms of client outcomes. These researchers describe caring as client-subjective experiences and/or physical outcomes after receiving actions or behaviors indicating that caring is present. Interestingly, behaviors deemed as caring by clients are likely to be more instrumental in nature than the affective and expressive behaviors deemed by nurses as indicative of caring (Morse et al., 1991).

From their review, Morse et al. (1991) pose several questions. First, "Is caring unique to nursing?" Morse et al. note that nursing theorists disagree as to whether caring is unique to nursing. From the universal human trait perspective, caring cannot be placed exclusively in the domain of nursing at the expense of other helping professions. Yet how caring might be uniquely manifested in nursing is not well delineated. Second, "Does the caring intent of nursing vary?" Morse et al. note that this question asks whether caring is constant or fluctuates depending upon the caring context. Most theorists agree that visible caring is variable, but on the philosophical or moral level, caring is the underpinning of the profession and must be stable, regardless of how a nurse feels personally about a client. And third, "Can caring be reduced to behavioral tasks?" Morse et al. note that scholars are in disagreement about this question as well. Obviously, proponents of perspectives seeing caring as a human trait, an affect, a moral imperative, or interpersonal relationships believe that caring is more than just skill or task proficiency. These scholars believe that the compassion and empathetic feelings of the nurse are requisite for clients to feel cared for. However, proponents of caring as therapeutic interventions and client outcomes believe that caring actions and outcomes do not occur unless caring is assumed to be present.

Perhaps another question is a dual one: "Does the expressively caring but unskilled nurse provide caring; and does the skilled but emotionally cold nurse provide caring?" The dichotomy in this question is apparent in the literature, with contrasting viewpoints such as that of Leininger (1991), who describes how the increased focus on the medical model and the introduction of technology in nursing beginning in the 1950s took away much of the humanistic focus on care, and that of others (Locsin, 2005; Mustard, 2002), who argue that simply having a caring ethos is insufficient to meet nursing's social and moral contract. Morse et al. (1991) recommend additional research to test possible theoretical links among the perspectives described. Such research may provide the empirical evidence needed to provide a more holistic, and possibly more accurate, understanding of caring.

Swanson (1999) provides the second important meta-analysis. In contrast to Morse et al. (1990, 1991) and to papers presented at conferences on the topic of caring, Swanson focuses less on the "philosophical underpinnings or importance of caring" (p. 32) and more on empirical data in order to provide a framework of care. In examining 130 qualitative and quantitative studies published between 1980 and 1996, Swanson proposes five levels of caring. These levels describe a process of caring that incorporates the various perspectives on caring mentioned earlier. However, Swanson ties them together into one framework. Swanson's levels include the capacity for caring, concerns/commitments of caring, conditions for caring, caring actions, and caring consequences. Swanson notes that these levels of caring

> are considered hierarchical not in order of import but in order of level of assumption. For example, an observational study of caring actions (Level IV) assumes that the individual or group studied had the capacity for caring (Level I), the commitment to act in a caring manner (Level II), and the conditions in place supportive of caring practices (Level III). (p. 33)

Within each level, Swanson notes that the literature further delineates characteristics or sublevels. For example, in Level I, "the capacity for caring," caring characteristics include being compassionate, empathetic, and knowledgeable, having a positive outlook, and being reflective. In Level III, "conditions for caring," there are various conditions that are related to the patient, to the nurse, and to the organization.

Although the framework proposed by Swanson (1999) is practical in its process-focused approach, Swanson contends that a great deal of research, particularly quantitative research, is needed to further delineate the levels and their interrelationships. In addition, Swanson notes that relationships between nurse and client are poorly represented in this framework. It is not clear which relationships would be considered caring and which would be considered noncaring. Although the framework is a representation of the current knowledge base and serves as an end-product model, important limitations are evident with regard to the framework and its hierarchical assumptions. For example, in terms of capacity for caring, how many of the listed characteristics must be present for caring to occur? If a nurse is knowledgeable and compassionate but lacks a positive outlook or reflection, has the nurse realized a capacity to care? In terms of assumptions, is it possible that caring actions can occur in an environment conducive to care and from a nurse committed to provide care, although this nurse is motivated more by financial gain and duty than the listed characteristics of a capacity to care? Another limitation of the framework is its likely bias toward Western culture and toward the perspectives of women. And, since the meta-analysis focused only on the nursing literature, it is unclear how generalizable the framework might be to other caring contexts, such as informal family caregiving and other helping professions such as social work and education.

Since the meta-analysis of Morse et al. (1990, 1991) was published, other authors have attempted to clarify caring as a concept. Unfortunately, their attempts have only confused the picture, offering little in furthering the development of a conceptualization of caring that can be operationalized and empirically tested. Phillips (1993) argues that the overuse of the term "caring" as a synonym for "nursing" has placed a false emphasis on the emotive aspects of caring, further enhancing a false dichotomy between care and cure. This dichotomy has long been discussed in the nursing literature. Leininger (1991) asserts that although care can occur without curing an illness, curing an illness cannot occur without caring for the client, thus underscoring the importance of caring in health. Phillips (1993) notes that the care/cure dichotomy has historically been couched in gendered perspectives, with cure associated with masculinity and high value, whereas care has been associated with femininity and low value. Today, authors argue that there really is no dichotomy at all, that if we assume that both caring and curing are directed at improving the health of clients, then caring and curing are inseparably interwoven (Kottow, 2001; Phillips, 1993). Such an argument, although worthy of discussion, adds little in clarifying care as a concept. In fact, Phillips suggests dropping the term "caring." She argues that "If nursing is caring, then the term 'nursing care' is tautologous.... Nurses already have a word for [caring] in the context of health promotion—it is called 'nursing'" (p. 1558). In contrast, others advocate for keeping the term "caring" in the context of nursing, but they argue that modifications of the term will provide clarity (Clifford, 1995; Scotto, 2003; Sourial, 1997). Clifford offers the term "formalized caring" for nursing, as it better reflects the social role nurses have in meeting the health care needs of individuals. Sourial proposes the term "holism" as a substitute for caring, since "caring seems to be part of holism...and the word 'holistic' is more clearly defined, understood, and scientifically based [than caring]" (p. 1191). And Scotto proposes that caring be defined as "offering of self" (p. 290) and that caring be understood to include intellectual, psychological, spiritual, and physical aspects. None of these new terms and definitions is empirically derived. The terms arise out of reinterpretations of previous work, and thus, none of these authors provide truly convincing reasons to change previous conceptualizations of caring.

Paley (2001) takes this last point to a rather dour conclusion. According to Paley, the purported body of knowledge of caring has not been developed in a rigorous fashion. Instead, what is known about caring is nothing more than endless associations and lists of attributes. Each new contribution provides no challenge to previous contributions, thus creating an endless morass of nondifferentiated terms and conceptualizations. As a result, one cannot apply theoretical caring knowledge as there are no testable differences among the caring theories. Paley states that

> I have argued that most of this "what is known" [about caring] can be found in a thesaurus, and that the reason for this is that nursing's way of knowing, at least as far as caring is concerned, is approximately 350 years out of date. It is preparadigmatic.... It is a knowledge of things said, a chain of association and resemblance which is constantly extended, constantly repeated. It represents an endless project, whose monotony is matched only by its uselessness. (p. 196)

Although Paley raises important concerns, he fails to provide an alternative approach to researching and understanding caring. Paley implies that nursing should just leave the concept alone, ignoring the multitude of studies and reports that clearly reveal the importance of caring, not only to nurses but to clients as well.

At this point, it is useful to return to Morse et al. (1990). Although these scholars acknowledge the historical confusion over the term "caring" and the need for further development, they do not advocate for the total disregard of the concept. These scholars note that progress is made as nursing moves away from the perspective that caring is simply a trait or moral stance within the nurse and toward a perspective that links nurse-centered attributes to realities that are client centered. In other words, if caring improves client health outcomes, then caring is a useful concept for nursing, worthy of further study and development. If caring is shown to be irrelevant to client outcomes, then nursing should no longer use it as a foundational component of a theory of nursing. Morse et al. propose that further examination may yield a new perspective, one that places caring as a component of a more encompassing, client-centered construct: comfort.

TRADITIONAL GENDERED PERSPECTIVES OF CARING

When caring is examined with the lens of gender, historically and pervasively caring has been associated with women and femininity. This association is strong not only in the nursing literature but also in the sociology and psychology literature. However, when caring has been examined in terms of gender, it is most often defined by its affective nature or as highly emotive with Madonna-like characteristics. Such a definition stems from traditional sociological theories, including a family division of labor perspective, in which women have historically worked in the home, providing domestic care to children and the sick and looking after the health of the family (Stoller, 2002). Men, on the other hand, worked outside the home and provided for the financial well-being and the protection of the family. It is not clear why general efforts to provide for and protect the family have not been identified as caring, especially since in nursing, providing for clients and protecting them from injury or health complications are essential. Freedom of choice and equity arguments aside, a question that comes to mind is whether the man who toils all day to exhaustion in order to feed and house his family is any less caring than the woman who toils all day to exhaustion in order to comfort and provide personal care to the children of the same family. Both types of work are essential to the success of the family, yet historically, it is the domestic work of the woman that has been identified as caring work. Continuing with this family division of labor perspective, men, with their work outside the home, have been afforded social opportunities not available to women in the home. These social resources are limited, however, so men have competitively struggled to obtain them. In such a situation, talent and/or power are needed to obtain resources and to maintain possession of them. Men with power may abuse it in attempts to weaken any possible competitors, including women who might venture out of the home or threaten male status. This abuse of power could be viewed as an antithesis of caring. For many scholars, the issue of power has become the central focus of study, with an examination of how men have been historically socialized to seek power and how men have used power to oppress others. This examination of power is not without merit. However, this focus has been one source of neglect of the recognition of the caring qualities of men. Other sources of this neglect include a lack of interest and the general acceptance that caring lies within the domain of women.

The assumption that men, with their drives for status and power, lack the caring qualities required of nursing originates perhaps most notably from Florence Nightingale, who advocated for the removal of hospital operations and patient care from the hands of men (Dossey, 1999). This assumption has contributed to the modern exclusion of men from nursing (see chapter 1) and has been the foundation for the numerous articles in the nursing literature warning of the dangers of increasing the number of men in nursing or introducing masculinity into the profession (for example, Ryan & Porter, 1993; Williams, 2001). This assumption was particularly strengthened by feminists, such as Gilligan and Chodorow, who tied caring to womanhood and not to manhood (Thompson, 2002), strengthening the premise that men are either inherently incapable of caring, or that caring from men only comes with great effort and at the expense of perceived masculinity. Going further, if men lack an inherent caring trait, they then lack the foundation for the use of caring as a moral imperative (Gilligan, 1982; Tong, 1993). Such assumptions, which result in definitions of caring that include only maternal and emotive characteristics, have greatly limited our understanding of caring. Such definitions can be likened to defining parenthood only as motherhood. In this scenario, if parenthood were taught to new parents, would children benefit if all parents provided only maternal love and no paternal love? Would society benefit from disregarding the caring associated with fatherhood? As silly as these questions might be, similar questions are implied by nursing's general lack of attention to possible, yet different, styles of care that men bring to the client's bedside.

If caring is a *human* trait, men also have the capacity to care. Boykin and Schoenhofer (2001) argue that "*all persons are caring* [their emphasis]. Caring is an essential feature and expression of being human" (p. 1). The ways in which this human trait or feature might be displayed in the emotional connectedness and the relationships men in nursing make with clients and the ways in which these affect the caring actions that men in nursing perform have largely been ignored by nurse scholars. In addition, no available empirical data examines the client outcomes resulting from possible masculine approaches to nursing care. (A few studies have examined clients' perceptions of the care they received from male nurses or their gender preference for the nurse [Ekstrom, 1999; Lodge, Mallett, Blake, & Fryatt, 1997]. These studies focused on gender and perceptions and not on the possible effects of gendered differences in the delivery of care.)

Though not mentioned specifically, the benefits of diverse styles of caring at the bedside are implied in nursing's recent call for the diversification of the nursing workforce. The exact styles that men bring to the bedside are not well understood. However, Morse et al. (1990) recognize general differences in caring styles and recommend further study of the topic. They state that

> The process of assessment and of styles of care is poorly understood outside the context of counseling. Nurses have the ability to adjust their approach and their style of interaction as they move from patient to patient.... For example, to the patient who is perceived to be suffering, the nurse's tone may be quiet and empathetic...to the young orthopedic patient, the nurse may be authoritarian. Delineation of these behaviors would be a significant contribution, yet to date these styles of care have not been explored. (p. 10)

MASCULINE STYLES OF CARE

So what might be a masculine style of care? On the one hand, this question is difficult to answer, since masculinity is itself amorphous. Masculinity is a fluid concept, one that is constructed socially and culturally from dynamic interactions with other individuals (Benyon, 2002; Bohan, 1993; Courtenay, 2000). As such, in any given social group, and within any individual, there are multiple masculinities that change as social contexts change. Given this caveat, however, there is some evidence that men in general conceptualize and implement caring differently from women. Within nursing, masculine care has scarcely been mentioned in the literature, as few have addressed the topic.

Two studies were located that focused on male nursing students as they learned how to care and reflected on caring (Paterson et al., 1996; Streubert, 1994). Both studies employed qualitative methods with small samples. Streubert notes that male students viewed their clinical experiences as an opportunity to apply theory to practice, develop clinical and team-building skills, and develop intuition. One student noted that it was imperative to develop an intuitive sense about a client's status, just as it is imperative to develop an intuitive sense about how well a piece of machinery is operating. In terms of gender, the students commented on the challenge posed by the societal expectations of men and the nursing context of physical and emotional intimacy with clients. Streubert states that this group of men was unique, and that "the intimacy with patients… is significant because it is available by virtue of their professional position as student nurses and not related to the establishment of a relationship over time" (p. 31). Paterson et al. provide more information on gendered differences in caring. From interviews with 20 male nursing students, Paterson et al. noted the emergence of the category "caring as male." These researchers report that beginning students did not identify gender differences in caring, but by the time the students had reached the junior level, gender differences were apparent to them. The junior students noted that women are socialized to care for others by freely showing emotions and touching clients, skills that came naturally to women but not to them. Several of the students reported feeling frustrated and tense since they were not sure they could easily adopt these feminine skills. By the time the students had reached the senior level, they reported that they had developed an amalgamation of what they perceived to be feminine and masculine styles of caring. The students identified masculine caring as the development of relationships with clients more akin to friendships than to the maternal relationship they perceived as developing between their female colleagues and clients. The students noted that male nurses were less "touchy-feely" than female nurses but had connections with clients that were nonetheless equal in meaning. Paterson et al. quote one student who said that he

> was amazed at the relationship he [another male nurse] had with his patients. He was loud at times. He told jokes. He teased them a lot. But they loved him. And you could tell he cared about them deeply. I think some of the female nurses on the unit thought he was too casual and not caring enough. I think they were wrong. (p. 32)

Another student observed that

> he [a male nurse] was sort of a friend, a tease at times, to the patients. He would go by their wheelchairs and give them a punch on the shoulder. It was a male thing. It wasn't the same as how female nurses cared for the patients, but it was caring nonetheless. (p. 30)

Paterson et al. note that, for the most part, male students had to discern gender differences on their own. The students reported that faculty members never discussed these issues with them, and expected them to care for clients as women would care for clients; faculty members were oblivious to the conflicts that might ensue. This perception was supported by an evaluation one student had received from his instructor about his approach to care, in which the instructor commented that he "needed to be more open with [his] patients...[and he should] watch her and try to be more like her" (p. 32).

This failure to address the issue by faculty was explored by the present author (O'Lynn, 2003), who surveyed 111 practicing male nurses who had attended 90 different schools of nursing. O'Lynn notes that 30.9% of the men reported that their nursing faculty had emphasized a feminine style when caring for clients. Of the 111 nurses, 46.4% felt that this emphasis constituted a barrier for male students. Interestingly, 53.6% of the sample reported that no masculine style of caring was presented to or discussed with them; and 56.0% of them felt that this lack of discussion was a problem. These findings suggest that the lack of attention given to masculine approaches is more common and more problematic than an emphasis on feminine caring styles.

Several studies included experienced male nurses in examining gender differences in nursing care (Gilloran, 1995; Ingle, 1988; Milligan, 2001; Watson & Lea, 1997). Ingle interviewed 12 male nurses about their approach to care. From the interviews, an overarching theme, "the business of caring," emerged. Ingle reports that this theme includes three categories with subcategories: supporting physical well-being (enacting skills, maintaining safety, surveillance); supporting psycho-emotional-spiritual well-being (being there, touching, listening, making eye contact, using facial expressions); and supporting individuality (advocacy and respect). Ingle notes that these men did not learn caring in nursing school, but rather entered nursing school with prior feelings and attitudes about care. It is not clear how the actions of this group of men may differ from those of female nurses. No further published discussion of Ingle's "business of caring" model was located. Watson and Lea developed a tool called the Caring Dimensions Inventory and tested its psychometric properties with 1,430 respondents, 34% of whom were student nurses and 11% of whom were male. Watson and Lea included 25 items on the tool, representing a rather limited list of nursing actions indicative of affective, instrumental, and teamwork tasks. Respondents were asked to determine whether or not each of the actions represented caring. Watson and Lea note that the men in the sample were significantly more likely than women to associate psychosocial tasks with nursing. It is not clear from the report whether or not these men were more likely than women to *implement* psychosocial tasks in their daily work. Gilloran interviewed 15 psychiatric nurses and notes that men tended to have more confidence and ability to make decisions than their female colleagues and were more concerned about career advancement. All the nurses welcomed a gender mix on the unit, describing the advantages of a diversity of perspectives. Again, little was said about specific differences in the delivery of care.

Perhaps the most informative study of male nurse caring was completed by Milligan (2001). Milligan interviewed eight male nurses and proposed a model of male nurse caring based upon the themes that emerged from the data. According to Milligan, male nurses view caring as meeting the biological and psychological needs of clients, working well within a team, achieving effective communication, and negotiating barriers to care. The anticipation of needs and the response to them are required in order to assist clients in gaining independence. With experience, male nurses adopt advocacy and concern for significant others as caring perspectives. Men learn to critique prescribed medical treatment that they feel is detrimental to the client's well-being. Men also develop a concern for the client's significant others and include them in communication and emotional support. This model lies within a societal context. According to Milligan, men are acutely aware that they constitute a minority within nursing and that some female clients may reject them as nurses. Men are also aware that societal expectations limit their emotionality despite the emotional labor required of nursing. Milligan expresses concern that these expectations may deter men from seeking support for the emotional labor they endure. The men also described the expectation that they provide physical strength to move clients or control aggressive clients, and the expectation that, as men, they will gravitate toward technical (and not emotional) tasks.

From these few studies, very little can be said about a masculine style of caring. The scholars mentioned above examined very small samples and provided very little, if any, comparison of their findings with existing theoretical models and perspectives of caring. However, these scholars provide limited support for the hypothesis that male and female nurses do employ different caring styles. These studies suggest that it is probable that men have the capacity and desire to care prior to coming to nursing. Men develop emotional interpersonal relationships with their clients and significant others, but they display this relationship with caring behaviors more indicative of a friendship than of a maternal, nurturing relationship. Caring is viewed as competency in anticipating and meeting client needs through nursing tasks, teamwork, communication, and advocacy. And perhaps masculine caring occurs within a social context that undervalues, and perhaps even denies, its existence, since it is not consistent with expected feminine caring styles.

It is possible that male nurses, after attending schools of nursing and working in clinical environments dominated by women and feminine styles, develop an amalgamation of styles (as noted above by a student), and thus they may not reflect a purely masculine style of caring. To address this possibility, one can examine the literature exploring nonprofessional caring contexts, such as family caregiving. Although a comprehensive summary of the caregiver literature is beyond the scope of this chapter, some points are particularly relevant. First, the findings from studies examining gendered differences in family caregiving are conflicting, due to methodological problems and/or gendered differences in self-reporting of psychosocial phenomena (Carpenter & Miller, 2002; Thompson, 2002). Second, few studies have proposed theoretical models of male caregiving, or fully described the experience of male caregiving in comparison with female caregiving. And third, most caregiver studies have examined the effect of caregiving approaches *on the caregiver,* and not on care outcomes as experienced by the care recipient. Thompson notes that traditional masculinity perspectives would suggest that men provide care from an emotionally safe distance, focusing on instrumental tasks rather than affective tasks. Such a conclusion has not been consistently demonstrated empirically, particularly when the prior relationship between the caregiver and care recipient is taken into account (Carpenter & Miller, 2002; Thompson, 2002). Thompson notes that men are more likely to adopt a "professional model" of caregiving, one that approaches care as work and focuses on task-completion, problem-solving, and the management of resources required to meet the needs of the care recipient. Such an approach may lead to less psychological stress on the part of the caregiver (Picot, 1995; van den Heuvel, de Witte, Schure, Sanderman, & Meyboom-de Jong, 2001). This professional model of care emphasizes control and compartmentalizes the burden of caregiving so as to prevent the caregiving from consuming the well-being of the caregiver. This model helps the caregiver temporarily forget about caregiver stress, so that the rewards and satisfaction gained from caring for and caring about someone increase. Thompson notes that some have described this approach as cold and uncaring, yet the evidence suggests that those who adopt this model focus on the needs of the care recipient more than on the societal role expectations of caregivers. Researchers have noted that many male caregivers, particularly husband caregivers, provide emotional nurturance in an amalgamated affective/instrumental fashion that blends characteristics of the professional model of care and emotive characteristics of care (Archer & MacLean, 1993; Harris, 1993, 2002; Hirsch & Newman, 1995). However, it is not clear how emotive nurturance from men may differ from emotive nurturance from women in a caregiver context.

Perhaps the professional model of care as described by Thompson (2002) is a pure form of masculine care. Perhaps the amalgamated affective/instrumental approach used by husband caregivers is akin to the amalgamated feminine/masculine style described by the nursing students quoted by Paterson et al. (1996). If so, then several questions come to mind. Is the pure professional model of care sufficient to communicate care, or is the amalgamated approach better in meeting objective and subjective client outcomes? Must men adopt an amalgamated style in order to become effective nurses? Does the adoption of an amalgamated style enhance a nurse's ability to apply caring approaches that are better tailored to differing care contexts? If so, should female nurses adopt an amalgamated style? These questions cannot be answered by the minimal amount of knowledge now available on this topic. Thus, additional research is needed. Answers to these questions would greatly enhance our understanding of caring as a phenomenon, would direct nurse educators to encourage male students with accustomed and/or comfortable masculine caring styles to apply them to client care, and, if amalgamation is preferable, would encourage female nurses to learn from their male colleagues as male nurses have learned from them.

THE ISSUE OF TOUCH

Whether or not men adopt an amalgamated style in providing nursing care, men must employ actions that address the affective needs of clients. But what do these actions look like for men? How "touchy-feely" must those actions be to meet client needs? More specifically, how do and should men touch? Touch is a caring behavior that has been a central focus in nursing. Touch is required to complete many tasks, but touch is also used to communicate caring feelings, comfort, and emotional attachment to clients (Estabrooks, 1987; Kidd & Wagner, 2001; Kozier, Erb, Berman, & Snyder, 2004; Leininger, 1991; Riley, 2004). However, touch is a behavior that is deeply defined by gendered and cultural rules (Evans, 2002; Leininger, 1991). How then do men negotiate touch?

Surprisingly in light of its importance to nursing, touch is poorly described in the contemporary nursing literature (Estabrooks, 1987). Estabrooks conducted a systemic review of articles appearing in the *American Journal of Nursing* and the *Canadian Nurse* published between 1900 and 1920 on the concept of touch, and compared these discussions of touch to those in similar articles published between 1970 and 1985. In the earlier articles, Estabrooks notes that there was much discussion of touch in terms of its use in procedures, as well as in promoting comfort for the client. Comfort uses of touch frequently occurred during bathing, massage, positioning, and the laying on of hands. This emphasis is also found in early nursing textbooks. Aikens (1928) states that

> Instinctively we feel that a nurse should be gentle, yet habitual gentleness requires a real effort and includes much.... The quality of touch is under our control. By the touch we may convey to the patient our

feeling of sympathy and tenderness, our appreciation of his weakened condition, our desire to be helpful. We reveal our character in our touch, to a considerable extent. (pp. 43–44)

Aikens continues:

> The comfort of the patients will be more entirely in her [the night shift nurse's] hands than on day duty.... Turning a pillow and shaking it for a restless patient, a gentle rub of the back or limbs, straightening wrinkles from the sheets...moistening parched lips...these are suggestions of comfort methods which need to be adapted to the individual patient, few if any of which will be included in the [physician's] orders. (pp. 113–114)

In contrast, Estabrooks notes, the comfort aspects of touch were notably absent from the later articles. Instead, nonprocedural touch was termed "affective" or "expressive." Such terms were used to indicate that touch communicated caring, but little was included on how, when, or in what context this type of touch should be employed.

This latter observation by Estabrooks (1987) was corroborated by the present author, who reviewed seven nursing skills textbooks commonly used today (Elkin, Perry, & Potter, 2004; Ellis, Nowlis, & Bentz, 1996; Kidd & Wagner, 2001; Kozier et al., 2004; Potter & Perry, 2001; Riley, 2004; Smith, Duell, & Martin, 2004). Within these texts, little content was provided on touch. Content focused primarily on the general benefits of touch, the assessment of the sensation of touch, and the fact that touch is interpreted differently in different cultures. No content was provided on how to provide touch, or specifically on how men should employ touch.

This lack of content on touch may be responsible for the lack of discussion that faculty members provide for male students on touch. Paterson et al. (1996) state that male students "reported feelings of confusion, resentment, fear, and embarrassment when they made first attempts to emulate touching that they had observed as 'female caring' " (p. 33). The students reported that the faculty did not understand what they were going through as they negotiated socialized masculine taboos regarding touch and the instructions they received to provide care with touch. Paterson et al. quote one student on this topic:

> They [faculty members] think that it is good enough to give us a lecture on the importance of touching. There were so many questions that I had back then. Like, do you touch everyone the same way or should you touch men and women patients differently? Or how do you know

> if a patient might not want to be touched or get the wrong idea if you
> touch them? (pp. 33–34)

The present author's own work supports the finding of the lack of content on touch in nursing school (O'Lynn, 2003, 2004). In surveying 111 male nurses, O'Lynn notes that 59% of nurses who had graduated from nursing school prior to 1992 reported that they had received no instruction on the appropriate use of touch from their instructors, and 68% of nurses who had graduated from nursing school between 1992 and 2002 had received no such instruction. In a follow-up study (results presented in chapter 9 of this book), O'Lynn reports that 49% of men who had graduated from four different nursing schools between 2002 and 2004 reported receiving no guidance on touch.

This lack of instruction is a serious problem for all nursing students, but particularly for men, since male gender roles in Euro-American culture severely limit the use of touch (Benyon, 2002; Evans, 2002; O'Neil, Helms, Gable, David, & Wrightsman, 1986). Violations of these roles put men in a suspect position. In addition, an increasingly litigious society and increased media attention and public awareness of sexual abuse and harassment have led to the belief that masculine touch is a vehicle for sexual advances (Evans, 2002). An example of this negative media attention is presented on Web sites that sensationalize the murders and rapes committed by men who are also nurses (Courtroom Television Network LLC, 2005). This societal context is evident in the comments of students who reported trouble with touch due to fears that a patient would interpret touch as seduction (Paterson et al., 1996).

O'Lynn (2003, 2004) also notes this fear in his study of male nurses. Of the men who graduated prior to 1992, 28% reported fearing false accusations of sexual inappropriateness while providing care to clients as nursing students, and 45% of the men who graduated between 1992 and 2002 reported this fear. In his follow-up study, O'Lynn noted that 34% of male graduates from four schools reported this fear. From this sample, there was no significant correlation between the age of the respondent and the presence of this fear. Interestingly, a majority of those who reported fears of false sexual accusations indicated that they *had* received guidance on touch. This unexpected finding suggests that it is likely that *the way* guidance is provided is more important than simply the provision of guidance. For example, if guidance is couched in terms of "don't do this" or "don't touch here," it is possible that male students will become more self-conscious about touch. Based on the finding, a search was conducted to see if any guidelines for nurse educators on how to guide male students on touching clients could be located. No such guidelines were located, so the following recommendations are based solely on anecdotal evidence:

1. *Innocent until proven guilty.* Nurse educators should presume that male students are ethical, professional, and entering nursing because they want to help people. Such a presumption fosters a climate of acceptance. In addition, when discussing touch, there should never be any implication that men are the responsible parties in "giving the wrong message." Misinterpretations arise from both parties. As such, men are not automatically at fault when clients misinterpret their actions.

2. *No requirement for automatic chaperones except in exceptional cases.* Policies that require chaperones for intimate procedures (such as postpartum assessments) negate the presumption of the student's innocence and good intentions. Automatic chaperones send a message that men are likely to be ill-intentioned or incompetent. Such a policy is also patronizing to female clients. Clients may wish to limit the number of eyes gazing upon their genitalia. As such, women should be asked whether they would prefer a chaperone or not. If a woman wishes for a chaperone, then one should be provided. However, chaperones may need to be provided automatically for clients who lack the maturity or cognitive skills to make such decisions or interpret intimate touch (such as children or clients with significant mental illness or dementia).

3. *Confidence with touch.* Although touch should be gentle, it should not be overwhelmingly light for most procedures. A weak touch communicates hesitancy and nervousness, signs atypical of a confident and competent professional.

4. *Touch accompanied by communication.* Students should be taught to notify clients, prior to contact, of when and where intimate touch will occur. In addition, casual conversation during intimate touch will help divert attention away from the touch and reduce stress for both student and client.

5. *Directionality.* Students should be taught "progressive touch." For example, during a urinary catheterization, the first touch should not be on the genitalia. Instead, with the nonsterile hand, students should touch a relatively safe area first, such as the knee. Then, the hand should touch the inner thigh while the student is informing the client about the need to touch the genitalia. The speed of the progression should be timed to the client's level of comfort, with slower, more deliberate progression if the client appears uneasy. While touching sensitive areas, the student should maintain contact with a less sensitive area. So during urinary catheterization, the elbow could maintain contact with the inner thigh or knee. Concurrent contact such as this reduces the intensity of solitary touching of sensitive areas. At the conclusion of the pro-

cedure, touch should be removed from sensitive areas as soon as possible.

6. *Privacy*. Naturally, students should allow for patient privacy during procedures by covering areas that do not need to be accessed and by pulling curtains. In settings where there are no curtains (as in a private room), the student should ask the client if she prefers to have the door completely closed, or left slightly ajar. Some clients may feel more vulnerable or cornered if doors are shut tightly.

7. *Cultural awareness*. Nurse instructors should review with students the general cultural considerations regarding gender roles and appropriateness of touch. Special attention should be given to major ethnic and cultural groups in the local area.

With experience, male nurses may become more comfortable with touch, and fears of false accusations may subside. However, these recommendations may continue to be useful for men. These recommendations have not been tested empirically. Investigations as to whether such education on touch will facilitate comfort and confidence for male nursing students are needed, as well as investigations as to whether such education will instill confidence in the students' performance from the perspectives of clients.

CONCLUSION

Although caring, as a concept, remains poorly understood, caring's importance to nursing is evident. Although proposed theoretical models of caring often appear to be inclusive of varied caring styles and approaches, traditional definitions and perspectives of care have limited the conceptualization of care to its affective aspects. These perspectives have associated care with women and femininity. Modern nurse scholars have done little to counter these limitations, as scant attention has been given to gendered differences in caring and care delivery. This creates challenges for men in nursing. Men come to nursing with gendered identities. The strengths and talents embedded in these identities are generally not encouraged in nursing. Still today, nursing gives the message to men that they must care for clients as women do, in order to be effective nurses. However, this message has no empirical support.

As men develop their individual styles of caring for clients, men may adopt what they perceive as an amalgamation of feminine and masculine approaches. Included within a feminine approach is the liberal use of touch as an affective action to communicate caring and possibly comfort. Touch is a highly sensitive issue for men, due to the cultural taboos against masculine touch and increased publicity about sexual misconduct. For many men, the need to touch clients (particularly female clients) must be balanced against a fear of false sexual accusations. The challenges of negotiating this balance are heightened by the lack of attention given to this topic by nursing faculty while men are in training. Recommendations have been provided to assist men in using touch in a confident and competent manner. Appropriate use of touch will communicate and demonstrate professionalism and caring to clients.

Most of the information regarding caring styles and touch provided in this chapter has very thin empirical support. Therefore, research is needed to delineate gendered differences in the delivery of care. Once this delineation is developed, investigation as to which clinical contexts are best served by which caring style or approach can proceed. It is likely that individualizing caring approaches to client contexts will improve outcomes, just as individualizing counseling approaches or individualizing wound management achieves better clinical outcomes. If such an assumption is corroborated, nurse educators must embrace, teach, and model diverse styles of caring. Preparing students to equip themselves with an abundance of diverse caring skills will improve the health of the clients we serve.

REFERENCES

Aikens, C. A. (1928). *Studies in ethics for nurses* (2nd ed., revised). Philadelphia: Lippincott.

Archer, C., & MacLean, M. (1993). Husbands and sons as caregivers of chronically ill elderly women. *Journal of Gerontological Social Work, 21*(11/12), 5–23.

Benyon, J. (2002). *Masculinities and culture.* Buckingham, England: Open University Press.

Bohan, J. S. (1993). Regarding gender: Essentialism, constructivism, and feminist psychology. *Psychology of Women Quarterly, 17*, 5–12.

Boykin, A., & Schoenhofer, S. O. (2001). *Nursing as caring: A model for transforming practice.* Sudbury, MA: Jones and Bartlett.

Carpenter, E. H., & Miller, B. H. (2002). Psychological challenges and rewards experienced by caregiving men: A review of the literature. In B. J. Kramer & E. H. Thompson (Eds.), *Men as caregivers: Theory, research, and service implications* (pp. 99–126). New York: Springer.

Clifford, C. (1995). Caring: Fitting the concept to nursing practice. *Journal of Clinical Nursing, 4*(1), 37–41.

Courtenay, W. H. (2000). Constructions of masculinity and their influence on men's well-being: A theory of gender and health. *Social Science in Medicine, 50*(10), 1385–1401.

Courtroom Television Network LLC. (2005). *Angels of death: The male nurses.* Retrieved November 22, 2005, from http://www.crimelibrary.com/notorious_murders/angels/male_nurses/index.html

Dossey, B. M. (1999). *Florence Nightingale: Mystic, visionary, healer.* Springhouse, PA: Springhouse Corporation.

Ekstrom, D. N. (1999). Gender and perceived nurse caring in nurse-patient dyads. *Journal of Advanced Nursing, 29*(6), 1393–1401.

Elkin, M. K., Perry, A. G., & Potter, P. A. (2004). *Nursing interventions and clinical skills* (3rd ed.). St. Louis, MO: Mosby.

Ellis, J. R., Nowlis, E. A., & Bentz, P.M. (1996). *Modules for basic nursing skills* (6th ed.). Philadelphia: Lippincott.

Estabrooks, C. A. (1987). Touch in nursing: A historical perspective. *Journal of Nursing History, 2*(2), 33–49.

Evans, J. A. (2002). Cautious caregivers: Gender stereotypes and the sexualization of men nurses' touch. *Journal of Advanced Nursing, 40*(4), 441–448.

Gilligan, C. (1982). *In a different voice.* Cambridge, MA: Harvard University Press.

Gilloran, A. (1995). Gender differences in care delivery and supervisory relationship: The case of psychogeriatric nursing. *Journal of Advanced Nursing, 21,* 652–658.

Harris, P. B. (1993). The misunderstood caregiver? A qualitative study of the male caregiver of Alzheimer's disease victims. *Gerontologist, 33*(4), 551–556.

Harris, P. B. (2002). The voices of husbands and sons caring for a family member with dementia. In B. J. Kramer & E. Thompson (Eds.), *Men as caregivers: Theory, research, and service implications* (pp. 213–233). New York: Springer.

Hirsch, C., & Newman, J. L. (1995). Microstructural and gender role influences on male caregivers. *Journal of Men's Studies, 3,* 309–333.

Ingle, J. R. (1988). *The business of caring: The perspectives of men in nursing.* Unpublished dissertation, University of Alabama at Birmingham, Birmingham, AL.

Kidd, P. S., & Wagner, K. D. (2001). *High acuity nursing* (3rd ed.). Upper Saddle River, NJ: Prentice-Hall.

Kottow, M. H. (2001). Between caring and curing. *Nursing Philosophy, 2,* 53–61.

Kozier, B., Erb, G., Berman, A., & Snyder, S. (2004). *Fundamentals of nursing* (7th ed.). Upper Saddle River, NJ: Prentice-Hall.

Leininger, M. (1991). *Culture care diversity and universality: A theory of nursing.* New York: National League for Nursing Press.

Locsin, R. C. (2005). *Technology competency as caring in nursing: A model for practice.* Indianapolis, IN: Sigma Theta Tau International.

Lodge, N., Mallett, J., Blake, P., & Fryatt, I. (1997). A study to ascertain gynaecological patients' perceived levels of embarrassment with physical and psychological care given by female and male nurses. *Journal of Advanced Nursing, 25*(5), 893–907.

Milligan, F. (2001). The concept of care in male nurse work: An ontological hermeneutic study in acute hospitals. *Journal of Advanced Nursing, 35*(1), 7–16.

Morse, J. M., Bottorff, J., Neander, W., & Solberg, S. (1991). Comparative analysis of conceptualizations and theories of caring. *Image: Journal of Nursing Scholarship, 23*(2), 119–126.

Morse, J. M., Solberg, S. M., Neander, W. L., Bottorff, J. L., & Johnson, J. L. (1990). Concepts of caring and caring as a concept. *ANS Advances in Nursing Science, 13*(1), 1–14.

Mustard, L. W. (2002). Caring and competency. *JONA's Healthcare Law, Ethics, and Regulation, 4*(2), 36–43.

O'Lynn, C. (2003). *Defining male friendliness in nursing education programs: Tool development.* Unpublished dissertation, Kennedy-Western University, Cheyenne, WY.

O'Lynn, C. E. (2004). Gender-based barriers for male students in nursing education programs: Prevalence and perceived importance. *Journal of Nursing Education, 43*(5), 229–236.

O'Neil, J. M., Helms, B. J., Gable, R. K., David, L., & Wrightsman, L. S. (1986). Gender-role Conflict Scale: College men's fear of femininity. *Sex Roles, 14*(5/6), 335–350.

Paley, J. (2001). An archaeology of caring knowledge. *Journal of Advanced Nursing, 36*(2), 188–198.

Paterson, B. L., Tschikota, S., Crawford, M., Saydak, M., Venkatesh, P., & Aronowitz, T. (1996). Learning to care: Gender issues for male nursing students. *Canadian Journal of Nursing Research, 28*(1), 25–39.

Phillips, P. (1993). A deconstruction of caring. *Journal of Advanced Nursing, 18*(10), 1554–1558.

Picot, S. J. (1995). Rewards, costs, and coping of African American caregivers. *Nursing Research, 44*(3), 147–152.

Potter, P. A., & Perry, A. G. (2001). *Fundamentals of nursing* (5th ed.). St. Louis, MO: Mosby.

Riley, J. B. (2004). *Communication in nursing* (5th ed.). St. Louis, MO: Mosby.

Ryan, S., & Porter, S. (1993). Men in nursing: A cautionary comparative critique. *Nursing Outlook, 41*(6), 262–267.

Scotto, C. J. (2003). A new view of caring. *Journal of Nursing Education, 42*(7), 289–291.

Smith, S. F., Duell, D. J., & Martin, B. C. (2004). *Clinical nursing skills: Basic to advanced skills* (6th ed.). Upper Saddle River, NJ: Prentice-Hall.

Sourial, S. (1997). An analysis of caring. *Journal of Advanced Nursing, 26*(6), 1189–1192.

Stoller, E. (2002). Theoretical perspectives on caregiving men. In B. J. Kramer & E. Thompson (Eds.), *Men as caregivers: Theory, research, and service implications* (pp. 51–68). New York: Springer.

Streubert, H. J. (1994). Male nursing students' perceptions of clinical experience. *Nurse Educator, 19*(5), 28–32.

Swanson, K. M. (1999). What is known about caring in nursing science: A literary meta-analysis. In A. S. Hinshaw, S. L. Feetham, & J. L. F. Shaver (Eds.), *Handbook of clinical nursing research* (pp. 31–60). Thousand Oaks, CA: Sage Publications.

Thompson, E. H. (2002). What's unique about men's caregiving? In B. J. Kramer & E. H. Thompson (Eds.), *Men as caregivers: Theory, research, and service implications* (pp. 20–50). New York: Springer.

Tong, R. (1993). Carol Gilligan's ethics of care. In R. Tong (Ed.), *Feminine and feminist ethics* (pp. 80–107). Belmont, CA: Wadsworth.

van den Heuvel, E. T., de Witte, L. P., Schure, L. M., Sanderman, R., & Meyboom-de Jong, B. (2001). Risk factors for burn-out in caregivers of stroke patients, and possibilities for intervention. *Clinical Rehabilitation, 15*(6), 669–677.

Watson, R., & Lea, A. (1997). The Caring Dimensions Inventory (CDI): Content validity, reliability, and scaling. *Journal of Advanced Nursing, 25*, 87–94.

Williams, C. L. (2001). The glass escalator: Hidden advantages for men in the "female" professions. In M. S. Kimmel & M. A. Messner (Eds.), *Men's lives* (5th ed., pp. 211–224). Needham Heights, MA: Allyn and Bacon.

CHAPTER SEVEN

Reverse Discrimination in Nursing Leadership: Hitting the Concrete Ceiling

Tim Porter-O'Grady

At a time when great strides in equality are being made and the strengthening of the value of the role of women in society has become a social priority, it is hard to believe that there is a subtle but clearly present inequity within the ranks of the largest group of professional women in the country. The role perceptions and expectations of men in nursing by women do nothing to dispel this inequity; indeed in many ways they facilitate it.

It would be inaccurate to suggest that this discrimination is intentional. Like most conditions of its kind it is quiet, unspoken, and insidious. Instead of being visually present in the consciousness of its holders, it lies just beneath the surface of the public persona of the discipline, where it operates with impunity, garnering very little attention (Diamant & Lee, 2002).

FOUNDATIONS OF REVERSE DISCRIMINATION

Reverse discrimination arises out of the same conditions as other forms of discrimination. Dependence, inequity, jealously guarded power, internal

A previous version of this chapter was published in *Nursing Administration Quarterly* (1995), *19*(2), 56–62. Reprinted with permission from Lippincott Williams & Wilkins.

competitiveness, and the maintenance of a relatively low position on the social hierarchy all drive the syndrome (Lester, 2002). When such factors exist in relationship to a specified group, they are enhanced within the group and also operate between the members of the group. When the opportunity to play out the behaviors of oppression on those that best symbolize the oppressors is presented, there is very little that can prevent internal oppressive behaviors from emerging.

The seven conditions that support this behavior are both classic and historic. They represent the foundations upon which the behaviors of discrimination are built in nursing:

1. Living in the shadow of a subordinating group, in which it is socially presumed that physicians provide the context and the parameters of behavior for nurses, substantiates second-class citizenship.

2. The restrictive licensing of nurses and the permissive licensing of physicians reinforce the limitations on the nursing discipline and its comparative narrowness of clinical judgment and functional activity.

3. The disparity in economic value between other major disciplines and that of nursing reinforces the limited value attached to the role of the nurse.

4. The traditionally held view that nursing is women's work, referring to the subordinating, delegated, cleaning-up ritualism of the work of nursing, retains a focus of mindless functionalism that belies intelligence.

5. The relative difference in socioeconomic membership in nursing as compared to medicine indicates a class difference between the disciplines, resulting in a different characterization of their members and their role in decision making.

6. The variety of entry points into the profession, which do not correlate with those of other disciplines, suggests that the content of the education of nurses is not substantive and, therefore, is of questionable value compared with that of other, more "rigorous" or well-regarded disciplines.

7. The lack of cohesion, collaboration, integration, and single-mindedness in the nursing profession reinforces the notions of separateness, competition, mistrust, and directionlessness that make its members easily manipulated and politically naïve.

These factors are present at varying levels of intensity between any and all members of the nursing profession. Men nurses do not experience these conditions any more widely than women nurses do. The weight of them, though, is more acutely defined by men in nursing than it is by their women colleagues. This happens simply because men can see the conditions' masculine origins. They cannot cope with the very male oppressiveness with which men burden women. Instead it is now directed at them, out of the very masculine paradigm that they themselves emulate. Men nurses are, in fact, being discriminated against on two fronts: by their own kind (i.e., other men) and also by members of their own profession (i.e., women). Indeed, the rules of relationship for men nurses are fraught with gender difficulties that often are not enumerated. This is especially true in leadership roles.

GENDER BIAS AND LEADERSHIP

It is expected, indeed reinforced, that men will ultimately choose to assume leadership roles in nursing (Group & Roberts, 2001). The expectation is reaffirmed by the notion that there is something wrong or suspicious about a man who appreciates and resonates with rendering good patient care and aspires to no other ambition. Even here there are degrees of acceptability with regard to the man's role. If the man works in high technology or in areas of high intensity or acuity, he is regarded as more acceptable than a man who prefers the more relational roles of medical-surgical or psychiatric nursing.

However, even for the man who may aspire to administrative or leadership roles, there is a sort of schizophrenia in the support given to him. While it is assumed as appropriate for him to move in the direction of management roles, any success he achieves in the venture is frequently attributed to the fact that he is a man and that he is somehow advantaged because of this. There is at times even a tacit indication that the fact that he does well in the role operates to the disadvantage of the women he may supervise. It is in essence a tale twice told: first, he is fulfilling the "natural" role for men and in doing so automatically disabling women who may be managed by him. Second, women are disenfranchised because the man holds the leadership position and, by holding it, prevents an equally qualified woman from obtaining it, thus tacitly reinforcing a root cause of gender inequity.

This reality also plays out in the politics of the profession. It is very challenging for men to break into what could be irreverently called the "old girl's club." Everyone knows how rarefied and sanctified is the "old boy's club" and how exclusionary it is to women and other "undesirables." This exclusionary politics operates in reverse but with just as much intensity in nursing. What makes it especially insidious is that there is no indication or intent, verbalized or acknowledged by nurses, to be exclusionary. It is simply that men do not come to mind when specific roles in leadership are available or national offices and special leadership opportunities for nurses arise. Even when the individual has made himself clearly available for such opportunities, the calls never come from those who are aware of his availability. This is not to suggest that there are no men in such positions. Each one, however, can tell a story of the challenges, including the effort necessary to achieve such a position, effort that must be made at a level of intensity not necessary for a woman in the same circumstances.

There are also examples of tokenism that often appear in the organizing of certain work groups, task forces, or other gatherings where it would be beneficial to be able to point out the inclusiveness and the diversity of members of the profession. Men, much like women in male-dominated professions, are included in nursing groups when it is apparent that to have a male presence is in the best visual or political interests of the group or of nursing.

The expectations of men and the problems these expectations create for men who are nurses are problematic for the discipline. In Great Britain, the expectation that men will provide leadership has frequently placed men in leadership positions at the expense of women. Only 10% of the nurses in England are men, yet they hold 50% of the leadership positions in that country. That is clear evidence that role expectations simply create an untenable situation that is difficult to change. While the situation is not quite as critical in the United States, men hold leadership positions in numbers that are disproportionate to the number of men in the ranks of nursing.

There is a potent, hidden disadvantage to the gender favoring of men in leadership roles: this relates to the use of the masculine paradigm for decision making and for constructing responses to the need for changes in the role and use of nurses in the service setting. The tendency toward male-based, linear techniques of decision making belies the greater need for the more appropriate feminine metatechniques for relationship building and for decision making. Masculinizing one more arena of health care will certainly advantage no one in the provision of health services; presuming that men are more naturally capable of management roles does nothing but facilitate masculine notions and techniques of leadership in the workplace.

At the same time, gender bias can disadvantage decision making when the contribution of men cannot be included in significant deliberations about policy, economics, and resource use, among other topics. In the current effort to construct meaningful health care reform, there has been a noticeable paucity of men nurses testifying on behalf of nursing and contributing to the conceptual shift in terms of what a nurse should be in the minds of legislators and policymakers.

As in the discussion regarding bias of any kind, it is hard to make a clear and cogent argument that describes with certainty the kind and intensity of the bias. Rather than being a clarion bell that rings for all to hear, bias is a muffled grunt that emanates from the discriminated in a wholly undifferentiated way. Since it is often so dispersed, it is hard to recognize and hard to obtain acknowledgment of it so that it can be addressed directly. It is often not readily apparent even to the one discriminated against until some time after the event, when further thought indicates to an individual that the circumstances don't appear to justify his exclusion from a role to which everyone would recognize he has a great deal to contribute.

ADDRESSING REVERSE GENDER BIAS

It must be pointed out that the profession of nursing is in transition from one kind of reality to another. The changes in the profession, especially with regard to role, parallel developments in the women's movement. As women become more equitably related to social institutions, there is a disproportionate emphasis on enhancing opportunities for women. This is especially significant when the normative fallout from such an undertaking is somewhat disadvantaging to men. This, of course, is true not just for nursing but for all the areas in which women have been actively seeking equal opportunities. It often appears that equity suffers as a result, and some of what ensues doesn't necessarily feel fair, especially to a person whose opportunities have been constrained.

The challenge for men in nursing is to recognize the existence of gender bias. While the majority of both men and women would like to believe it just doesn't exist, that would be naïve. On the other hand, it would be of no benefit to the individual or the profession to look for gender bias in all the circumstances of a career pathway. However, certain expectations related to the possibility of gender discrimination should be attended to and should challenge the male nurse to quickly provide an appropriate response. These expectations include the following:

1. Gender bias is often situational. If a situation or circumstance does not feel right and something appears untenable or disadvantageous, the individual concerned should follow up with questions related to the circumstances or situation until clarity is established to the individual's satisfaction.
2. If the bias is clear and certain, it should be not left unaddressed. If not dealt with, it is quickly repeated. Injustice and unequivocal

exclusion is inappropriate if not illegal, and the offended party
should not fail to take action.

3. A male nurse should anticipate the possibility of gender-related
    issues arising in the workplace. He might sponsor or teach a
    program on gender bias with a segment that deals with male
    recipient discrimination, so that this discrimination is made con-
    scious and people can visualize their own actions in relation to
    discriminatory practice.

4. A male nurse should clearly identify his personal expectations in
    relationships with others. He should let them know his sensitiv-
    ity to the issue and the arenas in which he most expects to be
    included, so that they are aware of what skill or contribution he
    might bring to the group and its work.

Men often come into the profession with the expectation that the
relationships they established in more male-dominated fields can pre-
vail in a female-dominated work arena. Nothing could be further from
the truth. The behavioral patterns in a predominantly female work
milieu are not the same as those in male-dominated environments.
Learning that lesson early in his career can help the man who is a
nurse navigate what could otherwise be a wholly negative experience.
It might be helpful to incorporate five realities into the mixed-gender
work profile:

1. Women value personal interactions and a higher intensity of
    communication than is often evident in a male-dominated work
    environment. What might appear as normative interaction in a
    primarily female work environment may seem excessive com-
    munication in many male-controlled situations.

2. Men are historically less in touch with how they feel than with
    what they think. This does not imply that women think less.
    However, their communication is more often expressive, com-
    pared with the emotionless communication found in many male-
    dominated environments. Women often display more interest in
    the meaning of an event or situation than in a purely dispas-
    sionate re-creation of the events as so often happens with men.
    An awareness of the impact of a statement or a behavior is as
    important in gender-mixed environments as the naked truth of
    the act or situation.

3. Traditional sociological development has led men to be quite
    comfortable with individual or collective competition. While
    competition may be just as evident among women, it is more
    subtle and less overt. Just as intense in female environments,

competition may not be specific or clear enough for some to visualize its presence. In such environments, the outcomes of aggressive or negative competition may often become apparent before an individual knows what was actually going on or just how it happened. Naïve individuals could pay a heavy price for their lack of awareness.

4. As in any environment, there may be those with a heavy dose of gender-based anger. For a host of reasons, these individuals seek opportunities to play out their anger on hapless and unprepared members of the opposite sex in an effort to make them feel as uncomfortable as the biased individuals do. The recipient of such anger may feel an overwhelming urge to pay the attacker back in kind, but that response rarely succeeds. Unless the one responding feels the same intensity of genuine anger, that person is totally outmaneuvered and can simply exacerbate an already untenable situation.

5. Sexual innuendo and sex-based jokes of any kind always stimulate gender-related discomfort. The content of the joke may well be harmless. However, when the workplace depends on mutuality, colleagueship, and equity in relationships, the introduction of sexual content may change the character of the interaction, relationship, and milieu. This, then, creates a new framework for interacting in the workplace and can lead to conversations, actions, or relationships that are inappropriate to a gender-integrated workplace.

SOME COUNSEL FOR WOMEN

A great deal of gender bias or discrimination can be eliminated by some simple evidence of role and relational sensitivity. Awareness and behavioral adjustment critically influence the kind of milieu in which men and women work together. Opportunities for the minority group can be facilitated by asking a set of simple questions. These questions are as follows:

1. In attempting to be inclusive in forming leadership or work groups, have you considered men nurses as a minority whose members should be recommended for leadership roles?

2. When opportunities for advancement are being considered, do you equitably look at the roles of all the players, including men, as you put together the potential leadership agenda?

3. Do you assess your own feelings about men in general when assessing the character of your relationship with them, so that you

can manage those parts of your bias that might be impediments to an effective relationship?

4. Is there evidence that opportunity in the organization is not gender specific and is inclusive and evidences representation from the full range of providers in the setting?

5. Has a mechanism been created to provide an opportunity to deal with gender bias and identify situations where it has been expressed, so that it can be dealt with in a way that satisfies potential complainants and raises consciousness within the organization?

6. Are there identifiable leadership cliques, indicating a need for a special relationship in order to advance in the organization, which effectively eliminates all opportunity for growth or advancement unless one subordinates oneself to the prevailing old boys' or old girls' network?

7. Does the leadership of the organization encourage and facilitate cultural diversity and programs that increase, specifically, the kind and number of nurses on important decision-making bodies in health care?

Answers to the above questions can serve to effectively evaluate the kind and quality of relationships that exist in the place where you work. While there are changing realities with new impacts on the workplace, there will be growing diversity both in gender and in culture. Old practices that limit opportunity for others based on any single factor not related to competence will prove to be increasingly unsuccessful. However, the opportunity for subtle discrimination never really disappears.

The challenge raised here relates to gender-specific activities, some of which exist in the most puzzling and insidious ways. The challenge to women in predominantly female environments sounds the same as the challenge that must exist in any other work context. Increasing sensitivity to individual interactions and relationships with men can often help clarify the need to make adjustments and reduce any exclusion that might result from failure to address the problems.

Inclusiveness does demand some conscious work with regard to what it means to be inclusive. Nurses do not always think of men when they are looking at political, organizational, or social advantages or opportunities. Nurses must cognitively acknowledge the need to be inclusive toward men in nursing just as is required with regard to any minority group. The richness and creativity of the contributions to the discipline and the delivery of health care can be enhanced through cultural and social diversity. In the case of nursing, that richness results from including men and effectively removing any impediments in the way of their using their many talents to continue to build an exciting and dynamic profession.

REFERENCES

Diamant, L., & Lee, J. A. (2002). *The psychology of sex, gender, and jobs: Issues and solutions.* Westport, CT: Praeger.

Group, T. M., & Roberts, J. I. (2001). *Nursing, physician control, and the medical monopoly: Historical perspectives on gendered inequality in roles, rights, and range of practice.* Bloomington: Indiana University Press.

Lester, T. P. (2002). *Gender nonconformity, race, and sexuality: Charting the connections.* Madison: University of Wisconsin Press.

CHAPTER EIGHT

Leadership: How to Achieve Success in Nursing Organizations

Daniel J. Pesut

INTRODUCTION

The purpose of this chapter is to identify principles and strategies that lead to successful leadership in organizational contexts. As the numbers of men in the nursing profession increase, opportunities for service and leadership in community groups, nonprofit organizations, and professional associations are open and available. Pursuit of leadership positions in organizational contexts is one way to focus one's values and realize one's purpose. Voluntary leadership and service through governance in professional organizations and associations enables one to influence policies and practices that are aligned with one's professional values, beliefs, identity, and calling. Service through leadership supports career advancement and leads to the development of talents and strengths. Leadership aspirations are often realized through involvement in communities of practice.

This chapter discusses principles that support successful leadership in organizational contexts. The decision to pursue leadership in a professional organization or association is often a function of personal talent, professional ambition, and organizational commitment. Through cultivation of personal strengths and talents, people often realize the importance of collective action to secure resources and serve a greater good. Understanding the basic governance responsibilities associated with service as a member of a board of directors and the characteristics of effective nonprofit community or professional association governance boards contributes to leadership success.

AWAKENING TO THE CALL OF SERVICE THROUGH VOLUNTARY LEADERSHIP

Consider the following facts about the numbers of people who volunteer and who engage in some type of service for the public good. Approximately 109 million adults (56%) are engaged in some type of voluntary social service. Volunteers contribute an average of 3.5 hours per week, totaling 20 billion hours with an estimated dollar value of $225 billion. Fifty-nine percent of teenagers volunteer an average of 3.5 hours per week, amounting to 13.3 million volunteers totaling 2.4 billion hours at a total value of $7.7 billion (Network for Good, 2005a). Volunteering creates new contacts, networks, and business, and personal and professional relationships. People also volunteer because it is meaningful and leads to the development of new skills. Some people volunteer because it helps them grow and develop as they deal with personal problems. For some, volunteering supports the development of communities of learning and practice (Network for Good, 2005b). Others volunteer because it helps them realize callings that help them manage their purpose.

Schuster (2003) states that "calls are invitations from life to serve, to activate your will toward a cause worthy of you and the human family. [Calls] are purposes with a voice, visions tuned into inner commands. Calls draw you into the specifics of a purpose and vision. A call is the impulse to move ahead in a meaningful way. It is a mind-body push into the future" (p. 34). Whatever your call, there are many opportunities in health care contexts to activate your nursing values and link them with the intention to serve and lead. Leadership and service contributions in professional or community associations are significant ways to serve and enhance the value of your call. Successful organizational leadership depends on personal ambition, as well as professional knowledge, skills, and abilities. In addition, understanding some of the expectations and responsibilities associated with the governance and leadership challenges in organizations is useful.

Realizing one's call and moving forward in response to such a call is one way to realize the good life. Leider and Shapiro (2002) define the good life as "living in the place you belong, with the people you love, doing the right work, on purpose" (p. 29). They note that many individuals have the following fears: the fear of having lived a meaningless life, of being alone, of being lost, and of dying. They suggest that work is the antidote to the fear of having lived a meaningless life. Love is the antidote to the fear of being alone. Place is the antidote to the fear of being lost. Purpose is the antidote to the fear of dying. Leider and Shapiro (2002) explain living the good life in this way:

> connecting our interests and desires to something bigger. This larger context can be made manifest through all sorts of approaches: a heightened sense of community, a commitment to the overall environment, a spiritual practice that places our own lives within a fuller perspective, even a sense of purpose from an organizational stand point. What's important is that we have a sense of place regarding the sources of our conception of the good life. While the manner in which we express ourselves is going to be highly individual, the central core of what we aspire to needs, it seems, to be grounded in something other than our own individual aspirations. We make the meaning of our lives, in other words, but that meaning apparently depends on something outside them. (p. 39)

Value is created when individual aspirations are connected with a greater purpose through service and voluntary leadership. Many individuals find that voluntary leadership through service within nonprofit organizations helps them manage purpose, helps them create and sustain relationships, gives life meaning, and provides a sense of place.

The philanthropic instinct associated with leadership commitments in an organization or community group is a special type of service. Individuals called to leadership through governance in professional associations or organizations find rewards as they aspire to higher standards of leadership. Nair (1997) concludes that a higher standard of leadership involves (a) a focus on responsibilities rather than rights; (b) an emphasis on values above policy; (c) respecting the service commitments made by self and by others; (d) an understanding of people emotionally rather than intellectually; and (e) the reconciliation of relationships between service and power. Successful organizational leadership requires attention to the details of a higher standard of leadership. Successful leadership in organizational contexts is also supported by personal ambition and professional knowledge, skills, and an understanding of the characteristics associated with leadership through governance. Based on my experience in organizations, I offer the following seven principles to consider if one desires to pursue leadership success in an organization or professional association:

1. Be intentional about voluntary service leadership aspirations.
2. Know your own signature talents and strengths and the ways in which they support effective leadership and governance in an organization.

3. Understand the power and value of alignment among logical levels in an organizational context.
4. Know how the governance process works in nonprofit organizational contexts.
5. Know how to be an effective board member.
6. Master the negotiation skills associated with competing values and polarities.
7. Understand issues of sustainability within nonprofit contexts.

These ideas and principles will be developed throughout the rest of this chapter.

Be Intentional About Voluntary Service Leadership Aspirations

Quinn (1996, 2002, 2004) suggests that one of the major dilemmas we all face in organizational life is the issue of slow death versus deep change. He notes that slow death is evident in an organization when people fail to anticipate and actively participate in personal, professional, and organizational renewal. Slow death is also influenced by the type of organizational lifestyle one chooses to embody. Quinn (1996) defines three basic organizational lifestyles: technical, transactional, and transformational. If one chooses a technical organizational lifestyle, one participates in and contributes to the technical success of the organization. Development of technical skills and competencies becomes a priority. Pride in technical competence is the aspiration. Personal survival is a key objective of a technical lifestyle commitment.

Commitment to a transactional organizational lifestyle requires more of a personal and professional investment. Curiosity, courage, and expertise in communication skills support a transactional organizational lifestyle commitment. With transactional commitment, individuals aspire to management roles and become concerned with the politics, interpersonal communication, and interpersonal transactions in the organizational context. Personal survival is still a top priority in this paradigm of organizational life, and it is achieved through attention to and influence on system politics. Transactional commitments require mastery of the art and science of compromise (Quinn, 1996).

The third organizational life style is what Quinn calls transformational leadership. Transformational leadership is built on the creative management of the tensions that exist between truth and vision, that is, the management of the gap between what is really going on in an organization and the organization's vision (Quinn, 1996). Transformational leadership requires a special type of consciousness and way of being.

Quinn (2004) contrasts a transformational way of being with our normal ways of being. He suggests that most of us live in a "normal" state of consciousness. A normal state of consciousness is one in which we are self-focused and ego driven. We put our own interests ahead of collective interests or relationships. We are externally directed. We define ourselves by how we think we are seen by others. We define ourselves by how well we obtain external resources. Quinn notes that in this state we are internally closed. We stay in our comfort zones. We ignore external signals for change. We engage in problem-solving activities. We are reactive rather than proactive.

An alternate reality or state of consciousness that Quinn associates with leadership is quite different. Intentional transformational leadership requires a state of consciousness in which we are focused on others. We transcend ego and put the common good first. This type of intentional leadership supports and encourages the development of connections and social-intellectual networks. Leaders are internally directed and strive to close gaps between values, beliefs, and behavior. Transformational leaders are externally open and move outside their comfort zones. They experiment to reach higher levels of discovery and develop competence. Leaders embrace deep change and commit to standards as they pursue meaning, purpose, and vision. Intentional aspirations for leadership move one beyond the technical and transactional model of leadership. Transformational leadership requires intention, effort, and commitment to deep-change work that is consistent with one's call and with the leadership contributions such a call demands. Thus, successful leadership begins with intrapersonal or inner work (Quinn, 1996).

Know Your Signature Talents and Strengths

Understanding and intentionally using one's strengths in an organizational context are among the keys to successful organizational leadership and governance. A strength-based approach to leadership requires knowing one's individual signature themes and natural talents. Buckingham and Clifton (2001) used Gallup Organization data from 1.7 million workers in 101 companies in 63 countries to craft the Strength-Finder survey. This Web-based survey enables people to discern their top five signature talents, strengths, or themes. Leadership success in an organization depends on being able to articulate the strengths and talents that one possesses and use those strengths in strategic ways to support the vision, mission, and purpose of the organization. Knowledge of strengths also supports the inner work associated with Quinn's (1996) notion of deep change. Having and using a vocabulary of strengths enables a person to understand his or her talents and skills and helps in the management of personal and professional purpose. Knowledge of one's individual talents and strengths accelerates understanding and action when one is involved in public organizations. The 34 Strength-Finder themes are listed in Table 8.1.

Many of these 34 themes tap into the important elements of governance models that work. Carver (1997) notes that good governance models must cradle a vision; thus, having a "futuristic" strength becomes important. Governance models also must explicitly address fundamental values and enable outcome-driven organizing systems, so maximizer, developer, focus, and connectedness strength themes are useful. In addition, governance also needs to produce forward thinking and separate large issues from small ones, and therefore strategic, learning, and input strength themes are valuable. Collectively, the talents of members of a board often enable an organization to excel through the diversity of individual strengths, if those strengths are known, valued, and appreciated.

TABLE 8.1   34 Strength-finder Themes*

Achiever	Futuristic
Activator	Harmony
Adaptability	Ideation
Analytical	Includer
Arranger	Individualization
Belief	Input
Command	Intellection
Communication	Learner
Competition	Maximizer
Connectedness	Positivity
Consistency	Relator
Context	Responsibility
Deliberative	Restorative
Developer	Self-assurance
Discipline	Significance
Empathy	Strategic
Focus	Winning over others (Woo)

* From Buckingham and Clifton (2001).

Understand the Power of Alignment and Logical Levels of Leadership

Leadership requires mastery of one's self; mastery of communication; mastery of relationships; and mastery of multiple ways of being, thinking, feeling, and doing in order to transform problems into desired outcomes. A variety of tools and resources support personal mastery and strengths-based leadership talent. A favorite leadership model of mine is the logical levels of leadership model proposed by Dilts (1996a and b). This model makes explicit the different levels and dimensions of issues that need leadership attention and influence. Dilts (1996b) suggests there are really three levels of leadership: the meta, macro, and micro levels. Metalevel leadership and change involves higher order attention and mindfulness to issues of community spirit and organizational vision, mission, and identity. Macrolevel leadership involves attention to pathfinding and culture building, and sensitivity to beliefs, values, and role configurations. Microlevel leadership involves attention to efficiency, task, relationship, capability, behavior, and environmental opportunities or constraints. When all of these levels are aligned within a person or within an organization, a high level of success results. When any of these levels are out of alignment then conflict, confusion, distress, and fear results. Leaders work toward alignment between, within, and among the logical levels in terms of the following issues: environment, behavior, capability, values and beliefs, identity, mission, vision, and contribution to the greater good within the community or systems in which the organizational entity functions.

The following questions help to make explicit the alignment of these logical levels. Armed with a knowledge of one's strengths, one can consider the following questions to discern an alignment between and among the different levels, as well as to determine congruence with leadership aspirations and strengths. These questions can also be applied to an organization, in order to quickly discern where levels of congruence and incongruence are located:

1. What is the *environment* in which you want to activate your strengths-based leadership? *When* and *where* do you want to use your strengths-based leadership knowledge? What will be the external context surrounding the strategic use of your strengths-based knowledge?
2. What are the specific *behaviors* associated with exercising strengths-based leadership? What, specifically, do you want to do in the contexts where you live and work? From a strengths-based perspective, what are the new behaviors you will develop that support your signature talents?

3. What *capabilities* are needed to meet your strengths-based leadership goals within the chosen context? How will you organize yourself to accomplish your strengths-based goals and behaviors? What capabilities or skills sets do you need to create/achieve your desired outcomes?

4. What *beliefs* and *values* are important to you as you consider your strengths and leadership goals in context? What motivates you toward leadership through service?

5. What role and *identity* level images come to mind in the context of your strengths-based knowledge? Who will you be if you engage those particular beliefs, values, capabilities, and behaviors in that particular context?

6. What is your mission, given the knowledge of your strengths and the contexts in which you operate? What are your strengths-based contributions to the *larger system or greater universes* in which you operate?

7. How does clarity about the greater purpose or vision you desire for yourself influence your identity, mission, values, beliefs, capabilities, and behaviors, and the environment in which you find yourself? (Dilts, 1996b)

Successful leadership in organizational contexts is supported by the alignment and understanding of the way in which each of these logical levels influences each successive level. Answering the questions posed above will help paint a picture of the many levels of commitment required for successful organizational leadership. One can also apply the questions to an organization and analyze relationships between and among the environment the organization finds itself in, the behavior of the organization, the capabilities, values, belief, identity, role, mission, and vision. Analyzing and evaluating relationships between and among these logical levels helps in discerning leadership strategies that support effective functioning and organizational success.

Alpha Leadership (Deering, Dilts, & Russell, 2002) is a model suggesting that three major leadership functions are anticipation, alignment, and action. Each of these functions includes a set of strategies that successful leaders use. For example, anticipation involves the detection of weak signals and the development of mental agility so that one can free up organizational resources to respond to innovations and new developments as they arise. Alignment builds on the logical-level questions noted above and includes the mastery of communication and self as one models leadership and relationship building in order to create cultures and organizations that can act. Action supports success as one strategically uses leadership strategies that accomplish aims and intentions.

Know How the Governance Process Works in Nonprofit Organizations

Various available resources provide information and guidance on the organizational governance of nonprofit boards; these include, for example, the works of Bailey (1989), Carver (1997), Chait, Ryan, and Taylor (2005), and Ingram (2003). Carver (1997) believes that most boards should focus on results or ends and leave the means to the chief executive officer (CEO) and staff of the organizations. Chait, Ryan, and Taylor (2005) suggest that governance is leadership when it combines attention to three modes of governance. The fiduciary mode is most operative when boards concern themselves with the tangible assets of the organization. The strategic mode involves creating strategic partnerships with management. The generative mode kicks in when boards focus less on remedial problem solving and more on creating the future through attention to different frames of meaning such as structure, human resources, politics, and the symbolic frame associated with the organizational culture, rituals, ceremonies, and expression of the spirit of the organization (Bowman & Deal, 1997).

When one examines the characteristics of effective boards, one begins to see elements of the fiduciary, strategic, and generative modes of governance in action. For example, Chait (2003) suggests that effective boards encompass six characteristics. Effective boards attend to the context and culture of the organization. Effective boards value education and seek opportunities to develop themselves and survey members to discern needs. Effective boards create a sense of community and inclusiveness among members. They groom future leaders and attend to all of the interpersonal issues that benchmark the successful development of community. Effective boards have analytic skills that help discern relationships among the complexities of competing issues. They value differences of opinion and seek out information that helps them in their deliberations. Effective boards are politically sensitive. Effective boards communicate with all stakeholders and attend to their needs. Effective boards are strategic rather than bound up in the day-to-day operations of the organization.

Ingram (2003) has developed a concise guide that outlines the 10 basic responsibilities of nonprofit boards. Successful leadership in an organization depends on board members being knowledgeable about their responsibilities. The 10 responsibilities of nonprofit boards are to do the following: (a) determine the organization's mission and purpose; (b) select the chief executive officer; (c) provide proper financial oversight; (d) ensure adequate resources; (e) ensure legal and ethical integrity and maintain accountability; (f) ensure effective organizational planning;

(g) recruit and orient new board members and assess board performance; (h) enhance the organization's public standing; (i) determine, monitor, and strengthen the organization's programs and services; and (j) support the chief executive officer and assess his or her performance.

Successful leadership in organizations depends on how well a board communicates the organization's vision, mission, and purpose to its membership and to the public. Vision and mission statements are crucial for setting the stage and making decisions about the allocation of resources and investments. Such leadership involves selecting, developing, and evaluating a CEO who works for the board. It is important to be clear about the differences between the board of directors' areas of responsibilities and those of the CEO. The selection of a CEO requires attention to the organization's vision, mission, and strengths. The development of a clear set of expectations and a position description for the CEO with well-defined parameters and executive limitations is one of the most important responsibilities of a board.

Providing financial oversight of the organization requires knowledge of fiduciary responsibilities. This requires attention to the budgetary process and to legal and accounting principles and practices, as well as attention to long-term financial strategies that contribute to the sustainability of the organization. One aspect of financial oversight is the value and importance of fund-raising and cultivation of donors to support the work of the organization. All members of a board have a responsibility to contribute to and develop resources that support the cause, mission, purpose, and vision of the organization.

Attention to the legal and ethical issues affecting the work of boards and associations is an ongoing board responsibility. Organizational policies and practices should be developed to ensure that ethical and legal vigilance receives attention. Records of the meetings and actions of the board need to be kept and archived. Conflicts of interest and commitment among members of the board need to be acknowledged. Published annual reports serve as a means to inform the association and constituencies about the activities and status of the organization.

Boards are responsible for planning and setting priorities in the changing environmental context. Most plans include attention to strategic directions of the organization built upon its vision, mission, and purpose. Planning often involves some assumptions about the future and about contrasts between current and potential programs and services. Such services are often predicated on the business plan and the financial support for initiatives. Communicating the plan to internal and external constituencies is a public relations function of the board and the organization as a whole.

Boards have a responsibility and obligation to seek out, recruit, cultivate, and orient new members of the organization and the board. This means that as a member of the board, one is always looking for people with new talents and with specific sets of knowledge, skills, or abilities that will enhance the work of the board or the organization as a whole. Part of this analysis should include periodic self-examination by the board as a whole, with attention to plans for board leadership and development.

As a leader in an organization or on a board, at all times, one is an ambassador for the organization. Clarity about organizational position statements and authority to speak the mind of the board are needed. Attention to communication plans and media training supports individual board members as they interface with community representatives, members of the organization, or public media. No individual member of a board should take it upon himself or herself to speak for the board or the organization, unless specifically authorized to do so. Clarity about how to enhance the public standing of the organization is an important ingredient of successful leadership in organizations.

The degree to which a board exercises its responsibility to determine, monitor, strengthen, and promote the organization's programs and services is a function of balancing member feedback with future planning, given the context of the organization's structure, resources, and governance mechanisms. Monitoring and evaluating program and service outcomes require skills in analysis and in asking strategic versus operational questions.

Finally, one of the major responsibilities of a board is the evaluation and assessment of the chief executive officer of the organization. The CEO works for the board and in many cases is its only employee. Evaluation is a process that supports and assists the CEO to perform more effectively. It is prudent to establish evaluation policies and procedures and invite the participation of the CEO in establishing the expectations and outcomes to be evaluated.

Attention to the collective responsibilities of boards as noted above helps ensure that everyone understands expectations. Making responsibilities explicit provides people with insight and understanding about how they can best contribute to the collective responsibilities of the board. In most instances, the board represents a unified stance in regard to decisions, actions, and directions. Individually, leadership success in an organization depends upon accountably following through with individual board membership responsibilities, which are discussed in the next section.

Know How to Be an Effective Board Member

An individual who commits to leadership in an organization or service on a board has individual responsibilities to consider. Consistently meeting individual board responsibilities contributes to one's success and to a reputation for responsible citizenship and leadership in the organization. The basic individual responsibilities of board service include attending meetings, participating in fund-raising activities, making monetary contributions, developing relationships, and negotiating conflicts.

It goes without saying that it is essential for individual board members to know the organization and its vision, mission, goals, and strategic directions. There are also duties of diligence, care, loyalty, and obedience that apply to individual board members (Bailey, 1989). Diligence requires that board members carry out duties with good faith and with the best interest of the organization or corporation in mind. It includes the creation and evaluation of programs, policies, and procedures that monitor the performance of the organization. A duty of loyalty requires that board members refrain from engaging in personal activities that would injure or take advantage of the organization. Any conflict of interest or commitment should be declared if it becomes apparent. It is important to serve the organization as a whole and to maintain independence and objectivity in deliberations, problem solving, and goal setting. Obedience requires that members of the board comply with the rules established by the governing charter of the organization.

Responsible preparation for meetings is a valued expectation for successful leadership. This includes understanding trends in the field and reading materials sent prior to meetings, as well as developing and asking questions that move discussions and debates along. The organization's financial statement should be closely read and understood in order to meet the fiduciary responsibilities of the board. Suggesting agenda items that need board attention is helpful. Undertaking or volunteering for leadership assignments or offering to assume the leadership of a board task force is an effective way to achieve success and demonstrate leadership. Maintaining the confidentiality of board deliberations or discussions in executive sessions of the board is essential.

It is helpful as a member of the board to support the CEO and behave appropriately at all times with the staff of the organization. A board member should not burden the staff with special requests for information or preferential treatment such as favors or special requests, should be clear about the boundaries between the board and staff in the organization, and should refrain from meddling in issues that belong to the CEO, who has supervisory responsibility for the operations of the organization.

Carver (1997) notes that in policy-setting boards, members of the board need to be clear about the ends they wish to achieve. The methods of achieving those ends are delegated to the CEO and the staff of the organization. This ends versus means distinction is a useful one for an individual board member to keep in mind. It is important to keep focused on the outcomes that the board and organization want to achieve. It is easy to fall into the trap of developing plans to get there. For some boards, this may be a comfortable way of operating. For others, plan development bogs the organization down and prevents the staff from using the full range of their knowledge, skills, creativity, and expertise in achieving the goals and directions established by the board.

Master the Negotiation Skills Associated With Competing Values and Polarities

Sooner or later, as a leader in an organization one is likely to confront the management of conflicts and/or polarities among members, organizations, or individuals that have competing values. Polarities exist in every situation. Tensions exist between fear and aspiration, the obligated and the entitled, scarcity and abundance, compliance and commitment, regret and hope, tolerance and prejudice, unifying and dividing, valuing and exploiting, illness and health, greater purpose and deepest fear, and slow death and deep change. Polarity management (Johnson, 1996) supports the development of creative systems thinking and community dialogue as people uncover the multiple dimensions, the upsides and the downsides, of polarized stances.

Polarity management contributes to successful leadership in organizations because it seeks to understand all sides of an issue or a stance. Johnson (1996) believes that if you take time to unpack a polarity, there are at least six ways you can begin to think about the issues embedded in the polarity dynamic. Johnson likens polarity management to breathing and he notes that organizations hire leaders to help the organization breathe! Consider a polarity involving tradition and innovation. If you have two camps, tradition bearers and crusaders, the members of each have a particular position they wish to advance. Most likely, the tradition bearers want to maintain the status quo and the crusaders want change. Each stance has some upsides. Each stance has some downsides. When these two positions are subjected to analysis that compares them with the greatest purpose of the organization and makes explicit the deepest fears of both camps, then there is room for dialogue. Strategic conversations can then be structured to work toward upside solutions for all, rather than causing everyone to be locked in an unproductive polarity debate.

Cameron and Quinn's (1999) work on competing values has a similar dynamic associated with it. An analysis of the literature revealed that most organizations get stuck due to competing values of focus and flexibility and of attention to internal versus external forces. Flexible organizations want to do things that are creative and externally oriented. Internally focused groups prefer incremental change and they focus more on controlling the change. Internally flexible groups, whose members understand the importance of building relationships through time, focus on collaboration and are likely to do things together. Successful leadership in this model involves alignment once again. The leader must align people, practice, and purposes within the context and matrix of the internal-external and flexible-focused preferences of people in the organization. These two models help leaders to be successful as they provide tools and strategies to negotiate the competing values and beliefs of disparate groups in organizations. Mastering negotiation skills with attention to polarity management and a competing values framework helps one understand how to meet both the individual and the collective responsibilities associated with organizational work.

Understand the Issue of Sustainability and Fund-raising for Nonprofit Organizations

Perhaps one of the most important elements of success for any organization is the degree to which it can acquire resources to support its sustainability through time. Successful leadership in organizational contexts requires attention to fund-raising and philanthropic efforts. Successful leaders contribute time, talent, and treasure. In many organizations, members of the board are expected to make monetary contributions through an annual giving campaign or a major gift campaign or through some type of estate or planned-giving program.

As members of a board, leaders are expected to provide both oversight and strategy to fund-raising efforts. Strategy is supported by attention to vision, mission, and the needs and programs offered and supported by the organization. Oversight is facilitated by the presence of fund-raising policies and procedures or, in some cases, a staff or foundation that has primary responsibility for fund-raising efforts.

Greenfield (2003) outlines some of the basic responsibilities associated with fund-raising by nonprofit boards. He notes that it is important to remember that fund-raising is always a voluntary activity. There are many ways organizations approach fund-raising goals. There are basically three types of giving in fund-raising efforts. These are annual campaigns and major or planned-giving options and programs. There may be other special types of campaigns or capital campaigns that are strategically developed to meet some goal or purpose.

In addition to personal giving, most leaders in organizations are invited to identify and cultivate relationships with donors and provide information to people who want to be involved in the sustainability goals of the organization. Donor contacts lead to donor growth, which in turn leads to donor commitment and investment in the organization.

It helps to remember that donors have their own aspirations and reasons for supporting the work of the organization. Fund-raising is easier when one can match a donor's aspirations with an organizational need or priority. Fund-raising success is dependent on the full participation of the organization's leadership. Board members are encouraged to identify and evaluate prospective donors and to cultivate and solicit gifts that actively support fund-raising programs. Support of fund-raising efforts through active attendance at functions and follow-up with donors is an expectation and part of the leadership responsibilities of board members. Members of the board are also responsible for evaluating success and ensuring ethical fund-raising practices among the board members and staff of the organization. Fund-raising is most often a new and undeveloped skill for novice board members. With practice and encouragement, raising money and finding ways to contribute to the sustainability and success of the organization become natural parts of a leader's skill set.

SUMMARY

The purpose of this chapter was to discuss seven principles associated with leadership success in professional organizations and associations. If you are interested in pursuing more formal preparation for leadership on national or international boards, consider applying to the Sigma Theta Tau International's Omada Board Leadership Development program. *Omada* is a Greek word meaning *team*. It is important to remember that leadership success in organizations depends on many talents and not just those of the leader. This educational experience is open to Sigma Theta Tau International members who participate in a structured 2-year board leadership development program. Participants are paired with a mentor and work with that person as they serve on a national or international board. For more information about the program or a list of references and resources used by the Omada program participants, you should visit http://www.nursingsociety.org/programs/omada_main.html. To learn more, read and review some of the references and resources listed at the end of this chapter. Achieving success through leadership is a worthy goal and may be one of the dimensions of your professional call.

REFERENCES

Bailey, D. (1989). *Directors and officers liability loss prevention for nonprofit organizations*. Warren, NJ: Chubb & Sons.

Bolman, L., & Deal, T. (1997). *Reframing organizations: Artistry, choice, and leadership*. San Francisco: Jossey Bass.

Buckingham, M., & Clifton, D. (2001). *Now, discover your strengths.* New York: The Free Press.

Cameron, K., & Quinn, R. (1999). *Diagnosing and changing organizational culture based on the competing values framework.* New York: Addison-Wesley.

Carver, J. (1997). *Boards that make a difference: A new design for leadership in nonprofit and public organizations.* San Francisco: Jossey Bass.

Chait, R. (2003). *How to help your board govern more and manage less.* Washington, DC: Board Source.

Chait, R., Ryan, W., & Taylor, B. (2005). *Governance as leadership: Reframing the work of nonprofit boards.* Hoboken, NJ: John Wiley and Sons.

Deering, A., Dilts, R., & Russell, J. (2002). Alpha leadership: Tools for business leaders who want more from life. New York: John Wiley and Sons.

Dilts, R. (1996a). *The new leadership paradigm.* Capitola, CA: Meta Publications.

Dilts, R. (1996b). *Visionary leadership.* Capitola, CA: Meta Publications.

Greenfield, J. (2003). *Fundraising responsibilities of nonprofit boards.* Washington, DC: Board Source.

Ingram, R. (2003). *Ten basic responsibilities of nonprofit boards.* Washington, DC: Board Source.

Johnson, B. (1996). *Polarity management: Identifying and managing unsolvable problems.* Amherst, MA: HRD Press.

Leider, R. J. & Shapiro, D. A. (2002). *Repacking your bags: Lighten your load for the rest of your life* (2nd ed.). San Francisco: Berrett-Koehler.

Nair, K. (1997). *A higher standard of leadership: Lessons from the life of Gandhi.* San Francisco: Berrett-Koehler.

Network for Good. (2005a). Participate in the tradition of volunteering. Retrieved July 7, 2005, from http://www.networkforgood.org/volunteer/volunteertradition.aspx

Network for Good. (2005b). 10 tips on volunteering wisely. Retrieved July 7, 2005, from http://www.networkforgood.org/volunteer/volunteertips.aspx

Quinn R. (1996). *Deep change: Discovering the leader within.* San Francisco: Jossey Bass.

Quinn, R. (2000). *Change the world: How ordinary people can accomplish extraordinary results.* San Francisco: Jossey Bass.

Quinn, R. (2004). *Building the bridge as you walk on it: A guide for leading change.* San Francisco: Jossey Bass.

Schuster, J. (2003). *Answering your call: A guide for living your deepest purpose.* San Francisco: Berrett-Koehler.

RESOURCES

Alpha Leadership: http://www.alphaleaders.com

Board Source (formerly the National Center for Nonprofit Boards): http://www.boardsource.org

Competing Values: Making Change and Innovation Happen: http://www.competingvalues.com

Network for Good: http://www.networkforgood.org

Sigma Theta Tau International: http://www.nursingsociety.org

CHAPTER NINE

Gender-Based Barriers for Male Students in Nursing Education Programs

Chad E. O'Lynn

INTRODUCTION

Currently, men comprise only 5.4% of the RN workforce (Spratley, Johnson, Sochalski, Fritz, & Spencer, 2001). Despite men's long history of working as nurses, men have been systematically discouraged from entering the profession. Although recruitment of more men into nursing could be accomplished by relatively simple marketing strategies, men cannot enter the profession unless they first enroll and complete their education in nursing schools. However, nursing schools frequently impose barriers for men (O'Lynn, 2004a). These barriers may result in higher levels of attrition for male nursing students as compared to their female counterparts (O'Lynn, 2004a; Sprouse, 1996; Villeneuve, 1994).

Keeping male students in nursing school through graduation clearly has important fiscal implications for colleges and universities. More importantly, however, reducing the number of men who leave nursing programs due to attrition or failure will increase the number of new nurses available to fill expanding vacancies in the profession as well as increase the overall diversity of the nursing workforce. These goals are important in meeting health care needs at present and in the future (American Association of Colleges of Nursing, 1997b, 2001; Anders, 1993; Buerhaus, Staiger, & Auerbach, 2000; Davis & Bartfay, 2001; Sullivan, 2000;

169

Villeneuve, 1994). This chapter will discuss the ways in which male gender serves as a source of barriers for men in nursing schools, review the results of a study examining a tool to measure these barriers, and provide recommendations for nurse educators and for further research.

GENDER AS A SOURCE OF BARRIERS

As any individual contemplates a career in nursing, a number of potential barriers must first be negotiated. Such barriers arise from financial or academic challenges, the bureaucratic hurdles inherent in academic institutions, time conflicts with current employers and family responsibilities, and personal anxieties and fears. These barriers often continue throughout a student's time in nursing school. The severity of these barriers and the ways in which they are negotiated vary among individual students. However, these barriers are not uniquely manifested in male or in female students. They have received much more attention in the literature than barriers associated specifically with male gender.

Much has been written about gender, how it is developed, and how it influences a variety of social phenomena. A comprehensive summary of the gender literature is beyond the scope of this chapter. Suffice it to say, some authors have noted that earlier perspectives on gender have focused on biological or socialization determinants (Bohan, 1993; Courtenay, 2000; West & Zimmerman, 1987). These earlier authors proposed an essentialist perspective on gender, in which masculinity or femininity are defined by specific characteristics or traits (Bohan, 1993). On the other hand, Bohan notes that a constructivist approach to understanding gender is better supported empirically. Constructivism assumes that gender is defined by the interactions people have with one another, in that these interactions have shared meanings as to what is appropriate and/or expected in terms of biological sex. In this perspective, gender is dynamic and active. Individuals negotiate gendered meanings on an ongoing basis with other individuals with whom they interact. Bohan provides a helpful analogy, noting that the differences between an essentialist perspective and a constructivist perspective are similar to the difference between identifying a person as friendly and a transaction as friendly. In the former, friendliness is a trait inherent within the individual. In the latter, friendliness is understood to be present according to the way in which an interaction occurs and progresses between two individuals as a result of the meanings of friendliness shared by the two.

Courtenay (2000) explains that gender is produced by dialectical and constructivist processes, resulting in a highly dynamic social structure. As such, persons have some influence on changing gendered meanings and on the ways in which gender is manifested. Courtenay states that

> From a social constructivist perspective...men and boys are not passive victims of socially prescribed roles, nor are they simply conditioned or socialized by their cultures. Men and boys are active agents in constructing and reconstructing dominant norms of masculinity. (pp. 1387–1388)

Viewing gender as an active, rather than passive, phenomenon has been proposed by others, such as West and Zimmerman (1987). These authors suggest that gender should not be viewed as a noun but rather as a verb. Gender is something people *do*, not something that people *are.* Consequently, people perform gender roles that manifest the perspectives (constructions), and their resulting behaviors, that originate from gendered shared meanings.

Gender is constructed variably, resulting in multiple types of femininity and masculinity (Beynon, 2002; Bohan, 1993; Courtenay, 2000; Thompson, Pleck, & Ferrera, 1992). However, people shape gendered constructions to be congruent with shared gendered meanings. Consequently, gendered constructions often result in norms that may appear at times to be static, hegemonic, and essentialist in nature (West & Zimmerman, 1987). It is important to note that a specific gender role developed and performed by an individual man is not constructed only from interactions with other men and male-dominated institutions but also from interactions with women and female-dominated institutions. Often, gendered meanings negotiated with other men are supported and reinforced by women. This is demonstrated overtly by the toys and leisure activities mothers provide for their sons, by adolescent girls' decisions as to which adolescent boys merit their admiration, and by the types of men preferred to grace the covers of romance novels and women's magazines. As will be noted, gendered constructions are reinforced within nursing by continued actions that feminize its imagery and language.

When shared meanings lead to gendered constructions that are relatively static and hegemonic in nature, individuals must engage in psychological and social labor and risk when they have to renegotiate those constructions due to life events or new social contexts. The increased intensity of these hegemonic forces increases the level of labor and risk. The conflict inherent in engaging in this labor and risk is described as "gender role conflict" and can lead to detrimental stress and behaviors (Good et al., 1995; O'Neil, Helms, Gable, David, & Wrightsman, 1986). Gender role conflict is defined as a psychological state where gender roles have negative consequences or impact on a person or others. The ultimate outcome of this conflict is the restriction of the person's ability to actualize their human potential or the restriction of someone else's potential. (O'Neil et al., 1986, p. 336)

Barriers, then, are structures and perspectives that reinforce hegemonic gendered constructions that result in gender role conflict. These structures and perspectives arise from interactions with one's family, peer group, and culture, as well as from interactions with social institutions, such as nursing academia. Since interactions vary greatly among individuals and over time, the influence a given barrier has on an individual is variable. It is of great importance that conflicts stemming from gender-based barriers may be lessened with actions that alter shared gendered meanings. Using gender role conflict as a theoretical foundation for understanding the unique barriers men confront in nursing school is advantageous, in that gender role conflict, as a construct, provides a better predictor and explanation of men's experiences and behaviors than other perspectives on gender roles and masculinity (Thompson et al., 1992).

BARRIERS FOR MEN IN DECIDING TO BECOME NURSES

As men consider nursing as a career, they do so with existing gendered constructions of nursing. These constructions may focus on nursing's assumed inappropriateness as a career for men, evidenced by the lack of positive male role models in nursing and the potential disapproval of family and friends. Traditional gendered constructions have even suggested that men who enter nursing are likely to be homosexual (Christman, 1988a; Haywood, 1994; Kelly, Shoemaker, & Steele, 1996), despite empirical evidence to the contrary (Christman, 1988a; Villeneuve, 1994). These constructions create a context in which barriers must be overcome in order even to submit an application to a school or college of nursing.

The influence on gendered constructions resulting from the ways in which the media portray nursing and nursing portrays itself cannot be overemphasized. For much of the last century, there has been a feminization of nursing's image (Christman, 1988b; Cummings, 1995; Davis & Bartfay, 2001; Villeneuve, 1994). Unlike professions that have traditionally been dominated by men, nursing has been slow to neuter its image. Despite recent media images such as those involved in the Johnson & Johnson advertisement campaign, in which men in nursing are positively portrayed, movies such as *Meet the Parents* (de Niro, Rosenthal, & Tenebaum, 2000) still portray men in nursing as misfits. Today, Florence Nightingale not only remains an important nursing role model but is seen as a symbol for nursing itself (O'Lynn, 2004b). Such reluctance to neuter nursing's image continues to reinforce the gendered construction that nursing as a career choice for men is aberrant. Although a few studies have indicated that young men may decide not to pursue nursing as a career due to nursing's perceived low pay potential or its high academic requirements (Barkley & Kohler, 1992; Villeneuve, 1994), aversive perceptions of nursing as a career for men remain evident in studies demonstrating that guidance counselors do not discuss nursing with young men (Barkley & Kohler, 1992; Kelly et al., 1996; Kippenbrock, 1990; Rochelle, 2002).

As a social institution, nursing is influenced by the sociocultural context within which it is embedded. However, the relationship is reciprocal. Nursing can influence the gendered constructions of itself that permeate society. Actions from nursing, such as protesting inaccurate and unflattering media portrayals of men in nursing, can facilitate progress in neutering the image of nursing. In addition, actions taken by individual schools of nursing can make a difference locally. For example, inviting local guidance counselors to an open house where they can learn about the opportunities for men in nursing has been shown to significantly correlate with increased numbers of applications from male students (Kippenbrock, 1990).

BARRIERS CONFRONTED BY MEN IN NURSING SCHOOL

If the gender-based barriers described earlier create a gender role conflict that is too great for an individual to overcome, he will likely not apply to nursing school. If, however, such barriers are surmountable or do not exist for an individual man, he will likely encounter another series of barriers that will exacerbate existing gender role conflicts or create new ones once he has become a nursing student. Most of these barriers are created by and/or influenced directly by nursing academia and individual schools of nursing.

The barriers actively set in place by nursing schools that challenge men come from two primary sources: (a) socioculturally influenced gendered perspectives on the appropriate behaviors and traits for men and women; and (b) the historical context of discrimination toward men in nursing. This discrimination has been described fully in other portions of this text, so it will not be detailed here. However, it is important to note that this type of discrimination generally subscribes to a loosely feminist perspective that nursing should remain feminized to counterbalance a patriarchal health care industry (Ryan & Porter, 1993) and/or subscribes to a fear that men in nursing will destroy either the unique qualities of a highly respected profession or that men will advance professionally on the backs of female colleagues (Evans, 1997; Ryan & Porter, 1993; C. L. Williams, 2001). Some people appear to combine gendered constructions and discrimination in a passive-aggressive fashion by stating that if men are to enter nursing, they should "do so on nursing's terms" (Ryan & Porter, 1993, p. 267), or that men should check their masculinity at the door upon entering nursing (as quoted by students, in Paterson et al., 1996).

From the literature, O'Lynn (2004a) identifies a number of gender-based barriers for men in nursing school. These barriers are described primarily in the findings of qualitative studies, reviews, and anecdotal reports, and can be roughly categorized as barriers related to (a) the feminine paradigm in nursing education; (b) a lack of role models and isolation; (c) gender-biased language; (d) differential treatment; (e) different styles of communication; and (f) issues of touch and caring.

The Feminine Paradigm in Nursing Education

In terms of the feminine paradigm, modern nursing education was born out of the model developed by Nightingale. Many nursing schools refused to admit male students well into the 1960s (Kalisch & Kalisch, 2004). Therefore, nursing educational pedagogy and theory have been developed and implemented from the perspectives of women for women. Evidence of this feminine paradigm is variable among individual nursing schools, but it is overtly seen in many schools' emphases on women's health content accompanied by a relative lack of men's health content; in the fact that there is little, if any, content on the historical contributions men have made to nursing; in an emphasis on feminist theoretical perspectives; and in the utilization of classroom strategies that are more advantageous to female learners.

Classroom strategies take on great importance when one considers the voluminous evidence that men and women generally incorporate different strategies for learning new and challenging material (Dunn & Griggs, 1998; Searson & Dunn, 2001). Although learning strategies vary among individuals, females tend to be auditory learners, who prefer quiet, formal classrooms, who are authority oriented, and who are motivated by parents or by themselves to learn. Traditional classroom environments favor such learners. These environments are not limited to schools of nursing, but they have particular relevance to nursing, which previously espoused values of obedience and servitude to authority figures. In contrast, males tend to be more visual, tactile, and kinesthetic learners, who prefer informal classroom environments characterized by mobility, action, and disruption, and who tend to be more peer motivated than females. In addition, males respond well to classroom debate of issues and to competition, as opposed to passive acceptance of the teacher's perspectives on the material. Although evidence in the nursing education literature supports efforts at diversifying the classroom environment, most male nursing students continue to report traditional, static classrooms (O'Lynn, 2004a).

The Lack of Male Role Models and Isolation

An important barrier for male nursing students is the lack of male role models (Kelly et al., 1996; Okrainec, 1994; Streubert, 1994). This barrier is strengthened by the small numbers of men in nursing and by the overall feminine imagery of the nursing profession itself. The visibility of role models can be enhanced by the inclusion of men in faculties of nursing, by the pairing of male students with male nurses in the clinical setting, and by the development of male mentorship programs.

Men are even more underrepresented on faculties of nursing than in the profession itself, with 3.5% of all nursing instructors being male (American Association of Colleges of Nursing, 2001). The importance of male faculty is noted by Kippenbrock (1990), who states that "The male students may perceive a closer collegial relationship with male faculty. They may also desire to emulate faculty. Possibly, they perceive the male faculty as being successful in a female profession" (p. 121). This perspective is echoed by Paterson et al. (1996), who note that students felt they could not discuss issues with female faculty members because they wouldn't understand and/or support a male perspective. These students also reported that they learned more from male nurses in the field than from female faculty members on how to negotiate gender conflicts surrounding communication, relations, and the use of touch. The lack of role models may lead some students to feel isolated, particularly from male peers (Kelly et al., 1996; Paterson et al., 1996). This isolation is further exacerbated by the time commitments required of nursing students and the general segregation of nursing students from the general college student body in many nursing programs. Strategies that may reduce this sense of isolation include mentorship programs for men, as well as liberalization of schedules to allow men to participate in general campus activities, such as fraternities and athletics.

Gender-Biased Language

In most societal circles, gender-neutral language has become the norm, so that terms such as chairman have been replaced by neutral terms such as chairperson. In regard to health professions, one rarely comes across the terms female physician or lady physician today. Yet the use of the pronoun "she" is still commonly used for the generic nurse in both text and conversation. In addition, the term male nurse is still used to describe a man who is a nurse, even when the biological sex of the nurse is irrelevant to the context of the text or conversation. Such language is bothersome for male students, who find it difficult to identify themselves in feminine terminology (Kelly et al., 1996).

The feminine imagery of nursing mentioned previously is also important in this context, since this imagery provides a nonverbal feminine language. Depictions of nurses as being only female create the same effect as the use of "she" for the generic nurse. Nonverbal feminine language is evident in the symbols nursing adopts for itself (such as the Nightingale oil lamp), in the teaching that empirical science is androcentric and disregards the perspectives of women (Campbell & Bunting, 1999; Duran, 1991), and even in the colors used in marketing programs (O'Lynn, 2004b; D. Williams, 2002). The use of feminine language and imagery creates an overarching symbol of how nursing identifies itself. Symbols create a common bond, a collegiality of sorts (Sullivan, 2000). When this symbol identification is overtly feminine in nature, men are made to feel uncomfortable and discounted (Sullivan, 2000).

Differential Treatment

The literature provides evidence that men receive differential treatment in nursing school, though most of the reports are anecdotal in nature. Much of the difference in treatment arises in situations where intimate contact is required between nurse and client. For example, many male students continue to report limitations placed on them in obstetric and pediatric rotations (Burtt, 1998; O'Lynn, 2004a), despite the lack of any evidence to support such limitations. Such limitations placed on men due solely to their sex create unequal learning opportunities, particularly when men are barred from client contact. In addition, such limitations reinforce the construction that men are unable to pursue, or are inappropriate for, certain nursing career directions. This construction creates a second-class status for men, a status that has been upheld in recent decades in some courts (Hawke, 1998). However, there is evidence that female gynecological patients with recent hospital and/or male nurse experience have no preference as to the sex of their nurse (Lodge, Mallett, Blake, & Fryatt, 1997), and neither do female obstetrical nurses with experience working with male nurses (McRae, 2003). Also, some students have reported being treated differently in practice labs. In such settings, it is customary for students to practice procedures on each other and/or on mannequins.

However, when intimate touch is required, men are often used as lab models, or male students (but not female students) are required to bring in an outside volunteer (Kelly et al., 1996).

Different Styles of Communication

The popular literature contains numerous books and articles that describe how men and women communicate differently. Chapter 5 is devoted to this topic. However, few nursing curricula address the communication differences between men and women, despite the importance of communication in workplace relations and interdisciplinary collaboration (American Association of Colleges of Nursing, 1998). Male students have reported that they struggle with communicating their concerns to female faculty (Kelly et al., 1996) and to female nurses (Streubert, 1994). Communication difficulties stemming from differences in style support the need for male role models and have implications in the classroom environment.

Issues of Touch and Caring

The use of touch is a major concern for students, but it is an issue that is rarely discussed by nursing faculty members (Paterson et al., 1996). These authors quote one student as reporting that

> the teachers never discuss it. They just think that it is good enough to give us a lecture on the importance of touching. There were so many questions that I had back then. Like, do you touch everyone in the same way or should you touch men and women patients differently? Or how do you know if a patient might not want to be touched or get the wrong idea if you touch them? (p. 33)

Male students reported anger with their instructors for not discussing touch and for not recognizing the discomfort they felt. Students reported that they had to navigate these waters alone, without a compass (Paterson et al., 1996). This discomfort is exacerbated when male students have gender-based limitations placed on them in clinical situations involving intimate touch. Disregard of the issue of touch enhances some male students' fear of being falsely accused of sexual inappropriateness when providing intimate care (O'Lynn, 2004a).

The issues surrounding touch impact the broader issue of care, since touch is a key and demonstrative element of human caring. Paterson et al. (1996) report that some nursing instructors have considered caring as an invisible (and thus, rarely discussed) construct for women because women are so familiar with caring behaviors. Male students report, however, that female faculty members and peers expected them to care for their patients as women would care for them. In other words, care was characterized by the heavy use of touch and emotionality (Paterson et al., 1995, 1996). Such an expectation creates a conflict for male students, who interpret these expectations to mean that they must behave like women to be proficient nurses. However, Paterson et al. (1995, 1996) note that male students were able to see that male nurses in the clinical setting employed caring behaviors that were not taught or modeled by female faculty. Such behaviors included the use of a teasing type of humor and a collegial (and nonhierarchical) type of interaction with clients and families. Male students felt that they were best able to learn how to care for patients from these male nurses. It is unclear whether female instructors do not recognize or do not value these possibly masculine approaches to care, and thus do not discuss them in class. The topic of gendered styles of caring is relatively unexplored in the literature. A more in-depth discussion of gendered styles of caring is to be found in chapter 6.

AN EXAMINATION OF GENDER-BASED BARRIERS IN NURSING EDUCATION

As already mentioned, gender-based barriers for men in nursing education have been described in the literature in qualitative reports, reviews, and anecdotes. However, O'Lynn (2004a) made an initial attempt to quantify the prevalence of these barriers and explore the perceived importance of them. Using the literature and anecdotes provided by male nurse colleagues, O'Lynn developed an inventory of possible gender-based barriers and submitted this inventory to a panel of nurse educators and deans for review. Adopting minor revisions recommended by the panel, O'Lynn developed a pilot version of this inventory (Inventory of Male Friendliness in Nursing Programs—Pilot, or IMFNP-P), in which respondents were asked whether or not a specific barrier was present and/or important in their nursing program. The IMFNP-P was mailed to 200 randomly selected male nurses, with a return of 111 completed surveys. Using descriptive statistics, O'Lynn noted that many of the barriers were present in the nursing programs of the participants, and that the participants reported that most of the barriers were important. Relatively few differences were observed between respondents who had graduated prior to 1992 and those who had graduated between 1992 and 2002. O'Lynn surmised that relatively few reductions in gender-based barriers had occurred in nursing education over the past few decades. None of the respondents recommended that additional gender-based barriers be added to the IMFNP, and none of the barriers met a priori criteria for removal from the tool. Thus, content validity for the items on the IMFNP was proposed. Upon completion of the study, O'Lynn (2004a) proposed a definition for a construct he termed "male friendliness" as a function of the perceived presence and importance of the barriers men confront as they strive to achieve academic success and satisfaction in their nursing education programs.

A proposition arising from this work and from gender role conflict theory is that male friendliness and gender role conflict have an inverse and reciprocal relationship. A consequence of decreased male friendliness and increased gender role conflict is increased stress among male students. This stress may help explain possible higher attrition and failure rates for male nursing students. This proposition is presented graphically in Figure 9.1. Strategies may be available for use by nursing programs to improve male friendliness and lower gender role conflict. However, future exploration of male friendliness and its relationships with other phenomena, such as gender role conflict, will require further psychometric evaluations of the IMFNP.

A FURTHER STUDY

Purpose

Although the pilot study identified no barrier that met a priori criteria for removal from the IMFNP, some of the barriers were deemed either *unimportant* or *neutral* by a majority of the participants. Although it is possible that the presence of numerous unimportant barriers on gender role conflict and stress might have a cumulative effect, it was determined that the presence of barriers described as *important* in the pilot study would produce a more demonstrable and conceptually sound effect. Therefore, the barriers deemed important by at least 70% of the participants in the previous study sample were included on the shortened version of the IMFNP (IMFNP-S). The purpose of the new study was to explore the internal consistency of the IMFNP-S.

Methods and Procedures

After ethics clearance was received from Montana State University–Bozeman, five nursing programs were recruited to participate in the study. These programs included one associate's degree program and four baccalaureate degree programs. Two programs were located in the Southeast

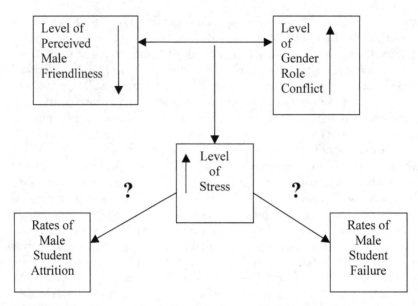

FIGURE 9.1   Proposed relationship between male friendliness and male student stress.

of the United States, one in the Midwest, one in the Rocky Mountain region, and one in the Pacific Northwest. These programs agreed to mail the study instrument to recent male graduates for whom they had current addresses and to current senior or graduating male students.

The study instrument used in the second study was the IMFNP, which had been used in the original pilot study but had now been revised, with a more discriminatory response set for each item. Survey items representing individual barriers were expressed as statements of presence, followed by a 5-choice Likert-scale response set ranging from *strongly agree* to *strongly disagree*. An example of a survey statement is as follows: "My program included content on men's health issues." Three items (presence of a mentoring program, male faculty, and other male students) contained only a *yes* or *no* response option. Numerous items were worded in reverse order, in order to prevent response set bias. Demographic information was also included in the instrument, as well as a form for qualitative comments about the tool. Instruction letters were included in the mailing, detailing the purpose of the study and giving assurances of confidentiality. Consent to participate was implied by the return of a completed survey. At the conclusion of the study, individual programs were given their own congregate results for informational and program evaluation purposes.

The rationale for using the IMFNP with all the original barriers (as opposed to the shortened version) was to provide the participating nursing programs with a full accounting of barrier presence in their institutions as per their request. Consequently, analysis of the data using descriptive methods was completed, with results from individual schools placed in separate reports and shared with the schools. For the main study, data from the IMFNP-S were abstracted from the IMFNP responses, for analysis. The analyses included descriptive and inferential statistical tests. Seventeen of the items on the IMFNP-S contained the Likert-scale responses as noted above. The scores for these items ranged from 0 to 4, with low scores representing high barrier presence, and thus, low male friendliness. Cronbach's alpha was calculated from the data from these 17 items using SPSS®. Two items (the presence of male faculty and the presence of other male students) were structured with *yes/no* responses. One point was given for the response of *no*, and three points were given for the response of *yes*. Since these items were dichotomous in nature, parametric statistical analyses were not used for them. The 19 barriers evaluated are included with the results, located in Table 9.1.

TABLE 9.1   Results from the IMFNP-S Study

Barrier (n = 78)	Mean	SD
1. Instructors referred to nurse as "she"	1.91	1.21
2. No history of men in nursing provided	0.78	0.01
3. No active recruitment for men to enroll	1.90	1.08
4. Faculty made disparaging remarks about men in class	2.31	1.21
5. No content on men's health	2.27	1.08
6. No opportunity to work with male RNs in clinical setting	2.17	1.29
7. Different requirements/ limits than female students in OB	1.96	1.30
8. No content on gender differences in communication styles	2.21	1.18
9. Not invited to participate in all student activities	3.05	0.88
10. Program did not encourage striving for leadership roles	2.81	1.07
11. People important to me did not support my career decision	3.31	0.74

Continued

TABLE 9.1   *(Continued)*

12. Felt had to prove myself because people expect nurses to be female	1.87	1.27
13. Male/female students treated more differently than expected	2.45	1.14
14. Gender was a barrier in developing collegial relationships with nursing faculty	2.54	1.14
15. Did not feel welcome as a man in clinical rotations	2.99	0.95
16. Nervous that female patients would accuse me of sexual inappropriateness from providing intimate care	1.92	1.17
17. Program did not prepare men well to work with females	2.10	0.08

Barrier	% Stating Present
18. No male faculty	34%
19. No other male students in graduation class	3%

Key: Higher scores represent higher levels of male friendliness due to absence of the barrier (higher scores are desirable). Scores for each barrier range from 0 to 4.

Results

A total of 170 surveys were mailed to men who had graduated between 2000 and 2005 from the five programs. A total of 78 completed surveys were returned, resulting in an overall response rate of 46%. The response rates for the individual programs ranged from 26% to 64%. The mean age of the respondents was 31.2 years (SD = 8.6 years, range 20–60 years), and 92% of the respondents were White. Thirty-four percent of the respondents reported that there were no men on the faculty while they were students, and 3% of the respondents reported that there were no other men in their graduating class.

The possible scores on the 19-barrier IMFNP-S ranged from 2 to 74, with the higher scores representing higher levels of male friendliness and a lower prevalence of important barriers. From this sample, the mean total score was 43.8 (SD = 10.3, range 13–66). Among the programs, the mean scores ranged from 39.8 to 51.4. Since only one program was represented by more than 30 respondents, inferential comparison of the mean scores among the programs was not completed. No significant correlation was noted between the age of the respondent and total score. However, respondents who had men on the faculty were significantly more likely to report higher male friendliness scores ($p < 0.05$).

One program was represented by 35 respondents. Using this program as a subsample, the internal consistency of the IMFNP-S was supported with a Cronbach's alpha of 0.80. Using the entire sample of 78 respondents, the internal consistency of the IMFP-S was supported with a Cronbach's alpha of 0.84. As with the original pilot study, none of the respondents recommended any additional gender-based barriers for further study. The results for each of the barriers on the IMFNP-S are shown in Table 9.1.

DISCUSSION

According to Nunnally and Bernstein (as quoted in Jacobson, 1997), for new tools, an alpha coefficient of 0.70 or higher is acceptable. As such, from the current study, initial support for the reliability of the IMFNP-S has been provided, and the IMFNP-S may be beneficial for use in future studies. However, for self-evaluation purposes, individual schools of nursing may prefer to use the full IMFNP in order to evaluate comprehensively the possible presence of gender-based barriers within its program.

In comparing the second study with the findings of the original pilot study (O'Lynn, 2004a), the ranking of barrier presence between the two samples was found to be remarkably similar, even though the second study's sample is much more homogenous than the pilot study's sample. Among the barriers that were included on both the IMFNP and the IMFNP-S, 8 barriers were identified by both samples as being among the 10 most prevalent. Both samples identified no content on the history of men in nursing as the most prevalent barrier, followed by the feeling that they had to prove themselves since people expect nurses to be female. This second barrier lends possible support to the proposed theoretical relationship between male friendliness and gender role conflict, as depicted in Figure 9.1.

It is important to note that the second study's sample includes men who completed their nursing education more recently than the men in the pilot study. Thus, the second sample may be more reflective of the status of barriers today. The second sample noted a lower prevalence of anti-male remarks made by faculty in class than in the pilot sample, and reported a higher prevalence of male faculty and male fellow students than in the pilot sample. These are positive shifts. However, the respondents in the second sample reported more frequently that they were nervous of being falsely accused of sexual inappropriateness when providing intimate care than did the respondents in the pilot sample. This finding is troublesome, in that it might reflect the growing need for faculty members to address issues of touch in a way that specifically meets the needs of male students.

The current study has some limitations. First, the sample size was small. Four of the five programs contributed fewer than 30 completed surveys, making an equivalency evaluation among the schools impossible. Second, there may have been a response bias. The characteristics of those who did not return a survey are unknown; however, there was variability in the responses in the sample. Third, the IMFNP-S contains only 19 of the original 33 barriers. This shortened version of the original tool may fail to reflect the perspectives of individual respondents who perceived less important barriers as being very important. And fourth, ethnic minorities were underrepresented in the sample.

It is recommended that the IMFNP-S be studied alongside the Gender Role Conflict Scale, in order to test a possible inverse relationship between the two constructs. If relationships among male friendliness, gender role conflict, and stress are supported empirically, a firmer theoretical foundation will be established for the examination of male friendliness and program outcomes, such as failure or attrition rates for male students. Such an investigation may provide evidence for the predictive validity of the IMFNP-S. A better understanding of how gender-based barriers might impair the success of male nursing students could assist education programs in developing strategies to enhance the male friendliness of its academic environment. Such a move is consistent with the directive from the American Association of Colleges of Nursing (1997a), which states that

> The objective for schools of nursing is the creation of both an educational community and a professional practice environment that incorporates the diverse perspectives of the many constituencies whom they serve…. Recognizing and valuing diversity and equal opportunity also means knowledgement, [sic] appreciation, and support of differing learning styles, ways of interaction, and stimulating forms of discourse derived from interaction and collaboration with persons from diverse backgrounds and experience. (para. 2–3)

It is not known whether many programs evaluate student outcomes in terms of gender. Since many programs have so few male students, it may be easy for faculty members to dismiss male student failure or attrition as being due to poor academic skills or discontent. Some in academia view their programs as testing grounds from which students with poor skills or bad attitudes can be weeded out, thus maintaining the integrity of the profession. However, when students are weeded out disproportionately by demographic category, such as gender, nursing academia must reflect upon its possible hidden or overt intolerance and its disregard of the call for diversification.

The directive quoted above does not necessarily create motivation for change in nursing academia. As with any bureaucracy, change can be immensely slow and painful. Perhaps the information reviewed in this chapter and the results of the second study will instill curiosity, motivating some to reexamine their programs. It seems, however, that individual critics and change agents must continue to challenge nursing academia to adhere to nursing's values of nondiscrimination and respect for individuals from all walks of life. Turning a blind eye to the unique needs and talents of male students is advantageous to no one. On the other hand, ensuring that the academic environment does not systematically advantage one group of students over another will improve nursing academia's ability to graduate a larger and more diversified student body ready to join the nursing workforce.

REFERENCES

American Association of Colleges of Nursing. (1997a). *Diversity and equality of opportunity.* Retrieved March 12, 2002, from http://www.aacn.nche.edu/Publications/positions/diverse.htm

American Association of Colleges of Nursing. (1997b). *A vision of baccalaureate and graduate nursing education: The next decade.* Retrieved March 12, 2002, from http://www.aacn.nche.edu/Publications/positions/vision.htm

American Association of Colleges of Nursing. (1998). *The essentials of baccalaureate education for professional nursing practice.* Washington, DC: Author.

American Association of Colleges of Nursing. (2001). *Effective strategies for increasing diversity in nursing programs.* Washington, DC: American Association of Colleges of Nursing.

Anders, R. L. (1993). Targeting male students. *Nurse Educator, 18*(2), 4.

Barkley, T. W., & Kohler, P. A. (1992). Is nursing's image a deterrent to recruiting men into the profession? Male high school students respond. *Nursing Forum, 27*(2), 9–13.

Beynon, J. (2002). What is masculinity? In J. Beynon (Ed.), *Masculinities and culture* (pp. 1–25). Philadelphia: Open University Press.

Bohan, J. S. (1993). Regarding gender: Essentialism, constructivism, and feminist psychology. *Psychology of Women Quarterly, 17,* 5–12.

Buerhaus, P. I., Staiger, D. O., & Auerbach, D. I. (2000). Implications of an aging registered nurse workforce. *Jama, 283*(22), 2948–2954.

Burtt, K. (1998). Male nurses still face bias. *American Journal of Nursing, 98*(9), 64–65.

Campbell, J. C., & Bunting, S. (1999). Voices and paradigms: Perspectives on critical and feminist theory in nursing. In E. C. Polifroni & M. Welch (Eds.), *Perspectives on philosophy of science in nursing: An historical and contemporary anthology* (pp. 411–422). Philadelphia: Lippincott.

Christman, L. P. (1988a). Men in nursing. *Annual Review of Nursing Research, 6,* 193–205.

Christman, L. P. (1988b). Men in nursing. *Imprint, 35*(3), 75.

Courtenay, W. H. (2000). Constructions of masculinity and their influence on men's well-being: A theory of gender and health. *Social Science & Medicine, 50*(10), 1385–1401.

Cummings, S. H. (1995). Attila the Hun versus Attila the hen: Gender socialization of the American nurse. *Nursing Administration Quarterly, 19*(2), 19–29.

Davis, M. T., & Bartfay, W. J. (2001). Men in nursing: An untapped resource. *Canadian Nurse, 97*(5), 14–18.

de Niro, R., Rosenthal, J., Tenebaum, N. (Producers), & Glienna, G., Clarke, M. R., Herzefeld, J., Hamburg, J. (Writers). (2000). *Meet the parents* [Motion Picture]. United States: Universal Studios.

Dunn, R., & Griggs, S. A. (1998). *Learning styles and the nursing profession.* New York: NLN Press.

Duran, J. (1991). *Toward a feminist epistemology.* Savage, MD: Rowman & Littlefield.

Evans, J. (1997). Men in nursing: Issues of gender segregation and hidden advantage. *Journal of Advanced Nursing, 26*(2), 226–231.

Good, G. E., Robertson, J. M., O'Neil, J. M., Fitzgerald, L. F., Stevens, M., DeBord, K. A., et al. (1995). Male gender role conflict: Psychometric issues and relations to psychological distress. *Journal of Counseling Psychology, 42*(1), 3–10.

Hawke, C. (1998). Nursing a fine line: Patient privacy and sex discrimination. *Nursing Management, 29*(10), 56–61.

Haywood, M. (1994). Male order. *Nursing Times, 90*(20), 52.

Jacobson, S. F. (1997). Evaluating instruments for use in clinical nursing research. In M. Frank-Stromberg & S. J. Olsen (Eds.), *Instruments for clinical health-care research* (2nd ed., pp. 3–19). Boston: Jones and Bartlett.

Kalisch, P. A., & Kalisch, B. J. (2004). *American nursing: A history* (4th ed.). Philadelphia: Lippincott Williams & Wilkins.

Kelly, N. R., Shoemaker, M., & Steele, T. (1996). The experience of being a male student nurse. *Journal of Nursing Education, 35*(4), 170–174.

Kippenbrock, T. (1990). School of nursing variables related to male student college choice. *Journal of Nursing Education, 29*(3), 118–121.

Lodge, N., Mallett, J., Blake, P., & Fryatt, I. (1997). A study to ascertain gyneacological patients' perceived levels of embarrassment with physical and psychological care given by female and male nurses. *Journal of Advanced Nursing, 25*(5), 893–907.

McRae, M. J. (2003). Men in obstetrical nursing: Perceptions of the role. *MCN American Journal of Maternal-Child Nursing, 28*(3), 167–173.

Okrainec, G. D. (1994). Perceptions of nursing education held by male nursing students. *Western Journal of Nursing Research, 16*(1), 94–107.

O'Lynn, C. E. (2004a). Gender-based barriers for male students in nursing education programs: Prevalence and perceived importance. *Journal of Nursing Education, 43*(5), 229–236.

O'Lynn, C. E. (2004b). A new symbol for nursing: An op-ed piece. *Interaction, 22*(3), 11–13.

O'Neil, J. M., Helms, B. J., Gable, R. K., David, L., & Wrightsman, L. S. (1986). Gender-role Conflict Scale: College men's fear of femininity. *Sex Roles, 14*(5/6), 335–350.

Paterson, B. L., Crawford, M., Saydak, M., Venkatesh, P., Tschikota, S., & Aronowitz, T. (1995). How male nursing students learn to care. *Journal of Advanced Nursing, 22*(3), 600–609.

Paterson, B. L., Tschikota, S., Crawford, M., Saydak, M., Venkatesh, P., & Aronowitz, T. (1996). Learning to care: Gender issues for male nursing students. *Canadian Journal of Nursing Research, 28*(1), 25–39.

Rochelle, R. R. (2002). *Recruiting men in nursing: Insights for the profession.* Unpublished master's thesis, Gonzaga University, Spokane, WA.

Ryan, S., & Porter, S. (1993). Men in nursing: A cautionary comparative critique. *Nursing Outlook, 41*(6), 262–267.

Searson, R., & Dunn, R. (2001). The learning style teaching model. *Science and Children, 38*(5), 22–26.

Spratley, E., Johnson, A., Sochalski, J., Fritz, M., & Spencer, W. (2001). *The registered nurse population March 2000: Findings from the National Sample Survey of Registered Nurses* (Report). Washington, DC: U.S. Department of Health and Human Services, Health and Resources and Services Administration.

Sprouse, D. O. (1996). Message from the president. *Interaction, 14*(3), 1–2, 4.

Streubert, H. J. (1994). Male nursing students' perceptions of clinical experience. *Nurse Educator, 19*(5), 28–32.

Sullivan, E. J. (2000). Men in nursing: The importance of gender diversity. *Journal of Professional Nursing, 16*(5), 253–254.

Thompson, E., Pleck, J., & Ferrera, D. (1992). Men and masculinities: Scales for masculinity ideology and masculinity-related constructs. *Sex Roles, 27*(11/12), 573–607.

Villeneuve, M. J. (1994). Recruiting and retaining men in nursing: A review of the literature. *Journal of Professional Nursing, 10*(4), 217–228.

West, C., & Zimmerman, D. H. (1987). Doing gender. *Gender and Society, 1*(2), 125–151.

Williams, C. L. (2001). The glass escalator: Hidden advantages for men in the "female" professions. In M. S. Kimmel & M. A. Messner (Eds.), *Men's lives* (5th ed., pp. 211–224). Needham Heights, MA: Allyn and Bacon.

Williams, D. (2002, Spring). Looking for a few good men. *Minority Nurse,* 22–28.

PART III

International Perspectives

What little has been written about the history and experience of men in nursing has focused on the West, and most recently, on male nurses in the United Kingdom, Canada, and the United States. This limitation may be due, in part, to the relatively large number of nursing journals and texts published in these countries and available through nursing databases and collections. In preparing this text, virtually nothing was located in the literature discussing men in nursing from Asia, Africa, or South America. Such a lack of information is important, since gendered experiences of men in nursing may differ among different cultures. In part III, Larry Purnell emphasizes the centrality of culture in gender manifestations and roles, and thus for men in nursing.

Due to the paucity of information on non-Western countries, part III provides only a small glimpse of men in nursing from an international perspective. It is hoped that it informs the reader that the challenges men face in nursing due to gender are not a uniquely Anglo-American phenomenon. It is also hoped that this section will inspire further exploration of the experiences of men in nursing across the globe.

—Chad E. O'Lynn

Gender-Based Barriers for Male Student Nurses in General Nursing Education Programs: An Irish Perspective

Brian J. Keogh and Chad E. O'Lynn

INTRODUCTION

The history of men in nursing in Ireland has not been widely document-ed, although several histories have been written about the Irish nursing experience. Men as nurses, in Ireland, have generally felt more comfort-able in mental health or intellectual disability programs, with few men entering general nursing education programs. General nursing education programs include content and clinical experiences in the medical-surgical, geriatric, critical care, pediatric, obstetric, and community health clini-cal domains; however, practice in pediatric and obstetric settings usually requires a postgraduate qualification. This position is mirrored in the United Kingdom, where men are more likely to be working in the mental health or intellectual disability branches of nursing (Finlayson & Nazroo, 1998). Although there is some literature suggesting that male nurses are confronted with a multitude of barriers, there is no empirical evidence that these barriers exist for Irish male nurses. This chapter sets out to describe the presence of perceived gender barriers and their perceived importance among male nurses who have undertaken the general nursing program in Ireland.

LITERATURE REVIEW

Nursing in Ireland has undergone radical changes in the recent years; the most notable of these numerous changes is the alteration in the way that nurses are educated. There has been a move away from traditional schools of nursing in hospitals to centralized universities in which full integration of nursing students with other college students occurs. In addition, the basic educational requirement for registration has become the bachelor's degree. What has remained constant is that there are three points of entry to the profession. Candidates entering the profession are educated to join the register in either the general, the psychiatric, or the intellectual disability divisions.

It has been suggested that men in nursing enter the profession for the same reasons as women (Lodge, Mallett, Blake, & Fryatt, 1997), and that men have historically been competent caregivers in a variety of settings (see, e.g., Mackintosh, 1997; Poliafico, 1998). The modern transition in which nursing became a predominantly female discipline has been attributed to Florence Nightingale, whose personal philosophy of nursing as a profession was purely a feminist one (Evans, 2004). Since Nightingale, there has been a steady decline in the recruitment of men into what is now perceived by the media and others as being a largely female profession. The belief that feminine characteristics are essential to nursing practice has led to the idea that not only is nursing a female occupation but also that nursing is somehow of low value in comparison to other, male-dominated disciplines, particularly medicine (Palmer, 1983). Despite greater efforts to reinforce the view that nursing is a profession with increased academic requirements for registration, negative views of nursing persist (Lyons & Petrucelli, 1978).

Recently, larger numbers of women have entered professions that were previously dominated by men. The same cannot be said for professions that are considered to be female dominated (Romem & Anson, 2005). Nursing continues to attract far more women than men. Interestingly, nursing has striven for diversity within its workforce, and active attempts have been made to attract people from a wide variety of ethnic, racial, cultural, and religious backgrounds into the profession (Sullivan, 2000). However, gender diversity is something that has not been adequately addressed (Sullivan, 2000), and only a token effort has been made to attract more men into the profession (Porter-O'Grady, 2003).

GENDER BARRIERS IN NURSE EDUCATION PROGRAMS

O'Lynn (2004) reports that much of the research literature on men's experiences in undergraduate nursing programs is qualitative and anecdotal in nature. From this literature and from interviews with male students and faculty members, O'Lynn has identified a number of potential gender-based barriers. These barriers identify challenges confronted by male nursing students in the following areas:

- The feminist paradigm in nursing education.
- The lack of male role models and the isolation of male students.
- Different treatment for male students during clinical placements.
- Different styles of communication among men and among women.
- Issues surrounding touch and caring.

O'Lynn (2004) constructed a survey tool, the Inventory of Male Friendliness in Nursing Programs (IMFNP), which queried respondents about the prevalence and perceived importance of possible gender-based barriers in their nursing programs. O'Lynn piloted the tool with 111 American male nurses and found that all of the suspected barriers were present to some degree, with each barrier having varying levels of perceived importance, as indicated by the study participants. Qualitative comments from the participants yielded no recommendations for additional barriers that had not been already addressed on the survey tool. O'Lynn noted that barrier prevalence was very similar among men who had attended nursing school within the past 10 years and those who had attended in previous decades, and suggested that gender-based barriers for male students are pervasive and have changed little over time.

O'Lynn (2004) notes that much of the literature he reviewed in developing the IMFNP came from the British, Canadian, and American literature. Since the historical, cultural, and structural aspects of nursing education may differ between the United States and Ireland, the application of O'Lynn's findings may be limited in Ireland. But since no similar study is available on this topic for Irish male nursing students, an exploration of the possible presence of gender-based barriers in Irish nursing programs is warranted.

THE STUDY'S AIM AND METHODS

Nursing education in the United States is very different from nursing education in Ireland. In the United States, unlike Ireland, all nursing students study the same curricular elements prior to taking a registration examination. After registration, nurses may elect to specialize in certain clinical areas through work experience, additional education, or both. This is important, in that all American male nursing students receive obstetric content and practice in their basic nursing program. As such, the barriers described by American study participants may differ from the barriers described by men enrolled in mental health or intellectual disability programs in Ireland, which do not include obstetric content and practice. Men enrolled in general nursing programs in Ireland would be most similar to the sample used by O'Lynn (2004). Therefore, the present study's aim was to explore the prevalence of gender-based barriers and their perceived importance to men who have undertaken *general* nursing programs in the Republic of Ireland. A quantitative paradigm was the methodological approach that underpinned this study.

A simple random sample was used to collect the data. An Bord Altranais, the Irish nursing board, generated the sample from male nurses who had completed a 3-year program in general nursing in Ireland. Due to the small number of men who undertake the program each year, a sampling frame was constructed to include all the male nurses who had completed the program within the past 10 years. Despite this, only 290 nurses qualified to participate in the study.

The questionnaire used in this study was an amended version of the IMFNP (O'Lynn, 2004). The original IMFNP was circulated to 10 male nursing lecturers at the researcher's university to be reviewed for its appropriateness for the sample. One IMFNP item pertaining to mentorship programs for male nursing students was omitted, since no such program exists in Ireland. Other changes made were more subtle, involving changes in wording or spelling to make the items more appropriate to an Irish sample. For example, the reviewers felt that the term "male friendliness" would be confusing for the participants. As a result of this specific example, the amended IMFNP was renamed the Inventory of Barriers to Men in Pre-Registration General Nursing Programmes, hereafter referred to as the amended tool or questionnaire.

The amended tool consists of 26 items that identify potential gender-based barriers for male nursing students and correspond to most of the items included on the original IMFNP. Each item is worded as a statement about the presence of a specific barrier. Respondents are directed to respond to each item with one of the following responses: *generally agree, neutral,* or *generally disagree.* Following each item is a question asking about the importance of the specific barrier identified. Respondents are directed to respond to each of these questions with one of the following responses: *important, neutral,* or *not important.* The responses to each item and the subsequent question indicate the respondents' perspective on the presence of a barrier in their general nursing program and the importance of a barrier. Several demographic questions are also included on the amended tool.

Following a small pilot study that tested the readability of the amended tool, the nursing board mailed the questionnaire to 250 participants, randomly selected from the sampling frame. Instructions were provided with the mailed questionnaire. The return of a completed questionnaire implied the consent of the respondent to participate in this study. The completed and returned questionnaires were analyzed using descriptive and nonparametric statistics.

RESULTS

Several questionnaires were returned to sender due to an incorrect address, or because the respondent was no longer practicing in Ireland. Exactly 100 completed surveys were returned, resulting in a response rate of 40%. The ages of the respondents ranged from 21 to 46 years, with a mean age of 30.5 years (SD = 6.2 years). The respondents had completed their training between 1996 and 2004, with the majority completing their training between 2000 and 2004 (n = 67). Just over half of the respondents had known a male nurse personally (n = 51), while only 31% stated that they themselves or a loved one had ever received care from a male nurse. Seventy-nine percent stated that there were male nurse teachers in the department of nursing where they completed their preregistration education. Just over half of the respondents felt that it was important to them as male student nurses that there were male nurse teachers present (n = 52), with only 15% stating that it was not important. The majority of respondents had between one and four other men in their graduating class (n = 82), and 12% had between five and nine men in their class. Six respondents were the only males in their graduating classes. A large number of the respondents (n = 79) felt that it was important to them that there were other men in the class, while only six felt that it was not important.

The results from barrier statements on the questionnaire are divided into two main categories: first, the reported presence of the barrier, and second, the barrier's perceived importance. The rankings of the top 10 barriers in terms of barrier presence are listed in Table 10.1. The rankings of the top 10 barriers in terms of perceived importance are listed in Table 10.2. For comparative purposes, the corresponding rankings from O'Lynn (2004) are also provided. The findings from O'Lynn come from the subsample of American male nurses who graduated from their basic nursing programs between 1992 and 2002 (n = 42).

TABLE 10.1   Rankings of Top 10 Barriers in Terms of Prevalence

Rank of barrier (Keogh) (n = 100)	% Stating barrier is present (Keogh/ O'Lynn)	Barrier (O'Lynn) (n = 42)
1 No history of men in nursing presented	90% / 88.1%	No history of men in nursing presented
2 No guidance on the appropriate use of touch	74% / 76.2%	Textbooks referred to the nurse as "she"
3 Textbooks referred to the nurse as "she"	74% / 66.7%	No guidance on the appropriate use of touch
4 No active encouragement as a man to pursue nursing as a career	72% / 64.3%	Instructors referred to the nurse as "she"
5 Different requirements limitations for male students during obstetrics placement	65% / 64.3%	No variation in classroom teaching methods
6 Instructors referred to the nurse as "she"	64% / 63.4%	Not encouraged to seek peer support from other male students
7 Felt had to prove self because people expect nurses to be women	60% / 53.7%	Felt had to prove self because people expect nurses to be women
8 Nervous that female patients might accuse student of sexual inappropriateness during caring interactions	57% / 52.4%	Different requirements limitations for male students during obstetric placements
9 Not encouraged to seek peer support from other male students	54% / 47.6%	Men portrayed as perpetrators of crime and not as victims
10 Anti-male remarks made by nurse tutors in class	53% / 45.2%	Nervous that female patients might accuse student of sexual inappropriateness during caring interactions

TABLE 10.2   Rankings of Top 10 Barriers in Terms of Perceived Importance

Rank of barrier (Keogh) (n = 100)	% Stating barrier is important (Keogh/ O'Lynn)	Barrier (O'Lynn) (n = 42)
1 Not feeling welcomed by staff during clinical placements	94% / 97.6%	Not feeling welcomed by staff during clinical placements
2 Nervous that female patients would accuse male students of sexual inappropriateness during caring interactions	92% / 92.9%	Nervous that female patients would accuse male students of sexual inappropriateness during caring interactions
3 Not including content on men's health issues during the pre-registration program	90% / 90.2%	Not being invited to all student activities
4 Decision to pursue nursing as a career not supported by important people in the student's life	88% / 90.2%	Decision to pursue nursing as a career not supported by important people in the student's life
5 No variation in classroom teaching methods	82% / 85.7%	Anti-male remarks made by nurse tutors in class
6 Not invited to all student activities	81% / 85.7%	No content on differences in communication styles between the sexes
7 No other men in nursing class	79% / 83.3%	Gender was a barrier in making collegial relationships with instructors
8 No opportunities to work with others on assignments and projects	78% / 78.6%	Not including content on men's health issues
9 Anti-male remarks made by nurse tutors in class	75% / 75.6%	Felt had to prove self because people expect nurses to be women
10 No active encouragement for men to pursue nursing as a career	74% / 75.0%	Not encouraged to seek leadership roles in nursing

DISCUSSION

Interestingly, the results of this study are remarkably similar to those of O'Lynn (2004), particularly when compared to the O'Lynn subsample of men who had completed their nurse's training recently. In terms of barrier presence, 8 out of 10 barriers were the same in both studies, with 6 of those 8 barriers identified by both samples within 10 percentage points. The similarities are striking, considering the cultural and structural differences between the nursing education systems in Ireland and the United States. It is possible that the similarities stem from the shared history these education systems have with systems established by Nightingale and her followers. Since many countries have nursing education systems based in this shared history, the generalizability of the barriers identified in this study is reasonable. Another possibility with regard to the similarities between the two samples is the pervasive feminist influence within nursing on an international level.

In terms of the perceived importance of barriers, there were fewer similarities between the two samples. However, both samples identified 6 out of 10 barriers that were held in common. Of these, 4 barriers were ranked within 10 percentage points of each other in level of importance. Several of the barriers that were identified as important by the participants encompassed issues concerning the socialization of men into the nursing role, for example, not feeling welcomed or not being invited to all student activities. However, the O'Lynn sample also identified barriers pertaining to professional development, such as leadership and communication. Importantly, the barriers described as important in these samples were identified as such by approximately 75% or more of the participants, suggesting that these barriers are of particular concern for male nursing students, regardless of whether these barriers were present in their programs or not.

Greater insight into these barriers is provided by the qualitative comments offered by the participants. The participants in this study were invited to provide general written comments at the conclusion of the questionnaire. Although O'Lynn (2004) reported that few of the participants in his study provided comments, many of the participants in the Irish study elected to provide comments. Most of these pertained to specific barriers identified on the questionnaire. For example, several participants commented on the need to prove that they, as men, were capable of becoming nurses. One participant noted that the "Disadvantages ... during my training and when I qualified, I [heard] that [men] were marked more leniently in exams and secondly we are lazy. Therefore, I tried to counter this by firstly being more academic and harder working than my female counterparts." Another participant noted that he discovered a misconception that male students were lazy and I felt that I had to prove myself that I wasn't one of these. Also, if you were ill or late on a Friday or any shift, it was suspected that you were in the pub the night before your shift. This was very stereotypical, as myself, I am a [teetotaler] ... and [am] offended by these comments.

Other participants commented on how they, as men, were sought out to relieve female counterparts of physical labor. For example, one participant commented that "Male nurses [were] seen as the human JCB for heavy purposes." Another noted that

As a student nurse, I was almost always asked to work in the area where patient dependency was highest, e.g., where the majority of heavy lifting was done. Also, I would often be called away from the area [where] I worked to assist with a heavy lift in another area.

These comments imply that some might accept male nurses for their physical strength, as opposed to other important attributes. Such a perspective becomes demeaning, as it harkens back to past times when men functioned in many facilities as untrained orderlies instead of professional nurses. The perception that men might be valued for physical strength over other nursing attributes indicates a possible barrier that was not addressed on the IMFNP or the amended tool. Future versions of the tool should perhaps include this topic as a new item.

By far the most common type of negative comment involved men's aversive experiences during their obstetric and/or gynecologic experiences. Overt discriminatory practices were described by several participants. For example, one participant noted that he was required to stand in the corridor when clients were assessed. Another noted that he was forbidden placement on the gynecologic unit, yet he was responsible for learning the same content as his female classmates, who all received gynecologic placements. One participant stated that "While on obstetrics placement, the majority of the female staff were hostile to male students, and those that were not hostile were decidedly cold." Another noted that the obstetrics placement was his worst experience. Such aversive experiences perhaps reflect long-accepted social mores. Although long-accepted, these mores are nonetheless discriminatory, as they do not apply equally to male physicians in these clinical settings. Although negative attitudes to male students on obstetric and gynecologic units may change in time, one wonders if nurse educators are implementing strategies to facilitate change. At least in the eyes of one participant, such strategies are nonexistent, as he noted, "Good luck with trying to change the system."

The role of the nurse educator in facilitating change needs to be stressed. Many of the participants noted that most of the negativity they experienced as male students did not come from clients or nurse tutors but from female classmates, female staff nurses, and female midwives. Negativity from these individuals is especially problematic for students. If nurse educators are problematic, students most likely have avenues for redress through the academic chain of command and/or grievance procedures. Problematic staff nurses and midwives in clinical sites are less likely to work in hierarchies that address complaints from nursing students. As such, male students may be forced to bear hostility based solely on their sex. As one student noted, men are expected to "just get used to it." Such hostility likely impairs learning. Since nurse educators bear responsibility for ensuring an optimal learning environment, ethical issues arise when educators place students in unfair and hostile learning environments without facilitating strategies to improve the quality of those learning environments.

Physical touching of intimate parts of the female anatomy is a component of obstetric and gynecologic care that conceivably leads to negative attitudes and behaviors toward male nursing students. Respondents in both samples noted that little guidance was provided to them about the appropriate use of touch. Since touch is a primary expression of care in nursing practice, it is puzzling that nurse educators appear to provide so little guidance. Men may feel unprepared to use touch, and, consequently, they feel poorly skilled at using touch appropriately when providing intimate care. This may result in compounded negativity from staff members in these units. In addition, this lack of preparation may lead to the increased fears that some men have of false complaints being made against them. Indeed, over 90% of the respondents in both samples identified fear of false accusations of sexual inappropriateness resulting from the provision of intimate care as an important barrier. O'Lynn (2004) suggests that this fear may be the result of an increasingly litigious society. However, Evans (2002) states that male nurses are often worried about false accusations that can ultimately affect their capacity to deliver the care that they are trained to provide. These fears may arise from societal beliefs that men who provide such touching are somehow deviant. This was echoed by one of the respondents, who noted that "Personally, we are not taken as professionals ... [but are] seen as predators, which of course is offensive at the highest order." Again, nurse educators can do much to alleviate these fears by instructing male students on how to use touch in a manner that exudes proficiency and professionalism.

Another issue identified by participants in both samples was the lack of attention to men's health issues and of the important role male nurses have had in the development of the nursing profession. Traditionally, histories of nursing place a strong emphasis on the feminization of the profession and the development of nursing as a female-dominated discipline in a decidedly patriarchal health care system. Mackintosh (1997) suggests that the failure to address the contribution that men have made to nursing leaves modern male nurses with little information about their historical roots and their professional backgrounds. She goes on to recommend that the contribution men have made to nursing history should be positively recognized; this would allow male nurses to contextualize their place as part of the nursing profession. Evans (2004) argues that, historically, male nurses have played an important but invisible role as nurses, and that this invisibility has perpetuated the idea that nursing is a woman's occupation, thus presenting a barrier to the recruitment and retention of men in the profession. Evans goes on to suggest that in order to improve recruitment and retention strategies aimed at men, the profession must acknowledge and understand these barriers and the ways in which they impact on men in the profession. Attention to men's health issues can be viewed similarly, in that such attention assists male students in placing their nursing role in their lives at a level of relevancy to which female students are accustomed, due to nursing academia's emphasis on women's health care. The high level of importance of men's health issues to the participants is evident in the findings from both samples.

Not all of the participants described gender-based barriers as problematic for them as individuals. Although they were in the minority, some participants provided positive comments. For example, one participant stated that "Most of the time, gender issues were not a problem." Another stated that "I didn't feel gender made a huge difference in pre-registration. I was treated very well."

RECOMMENDATIONS AND CONCLUSION

This study aimed to examine the existence, the prevalence, and the perceived importance of gender-based barriers for men who have undertaken general nursing programs in Ireland. In doing so, it has highlighted the fact that gender-based barriers do exist for men in Ireland preparing to enter the predominantly female nursing workforce. This is something that has not been examined previously, and thus the study provides an outline of the experience of male students during their registration training. The barriers provide additional challenges for male students that are not shared by their female colleagues, thus placing them at a possible disadvantage.

The additional challenges faced by male nursing students may impair their ability to complete their programs satisfactorily or may impair their socialization into the profession. Future research will be needed to evaluate how barriers might disproportionately affect the academic performance of male students. However, some evidence for the continuing effect of gender-based barriers was provided by a couple of participants in this study, who stated that they were planning to leave nursing. One participant noted that "Some of the barriers experienced throughout my training and since qualifying have, in part, led me to pursuing an alternative career."

The fact that barriers experienced as nursing students persist into men's careers is highly disturbing. Numerous sources have indicated that increased numbers of men are needed in nursing in order to provide workforce diversity (see, e.g., Porter-O'Grady [2003]; Sullivan [2000]) as well as to lessen the effects of the nursing shortage (Government of Ireland, 1998). It is clear that simply attracting men into nursing programs through marketing strategies or scholarships will not meet either the goal of diversification or the goal of increasing the size of the nursing workforce. The gender-based barriers experienced by men first as nursing students and then as clinicians must be addressed before recruitment and retention goals can be attained. Additional research is strongly recommended to further explore these barriers, their impact on academic outcomes, and their effect on the retention of men in the nursing workforce.

REFERENCES

Evans, J. (2002). Cautious caregivers: Gender stereotypes and the sexualization of men nurses' touch. *Journal of Advanced Nursing, 40*(4), 441–448.

Evans, J. (2004). Men nurses: A historical and feminist perspective. *Journal of Advanced Nursing, 47*(3), 321–328.

Finlayson, L., & Nazroo, J. (1998). *Gender inequalities in nursing careers.* London: Policy Studies Institute.

Government of Ireland, Department of Health and Children. (1998). *Report of the Commission on Nursing: A blueprint for the future.* Dublin: Author.

Lodge, N., Mallett, J., Blake, P., & Fryatt, I. (1997). A study to ascertain gynaecological patients' perceived levels of embarrassment with physical and psychological care given by female and male nurses. *Journal of Advanced Nursing, 25*(5), 893–907.

Lyons, A., & Petrucelli, R. (1978). *Medicine: An illustrated history.* New York: Harry N. Abrams Publishers.

Mackintosh, C. (1997) .A historical study of men in nursing. *Journal of Advanced Nursing, 26*(2), 232–236.

O'Lynn, C. (2004). Gender-based barriers for male students in nursing education programs: Prevalence and perceived importance. *Journal of Nursing Education, 43*(5), 229–236.

Palmer, I. (1983). Nightingale revisited. *Nursing Outlook, 31*(4), 229–233.

Poliafico, J. (1998). Nursing's gender gap. *RN, 61*(10), 39–42.

Porter-O'Grady, T. (2003). Where are the men? *Nursing 2003, 33*(7), 43–45.

Romem, P., & Anson, O. (2005) Israeli men in nursing: Social and personal motives. *Journal of Nursing Management, 13*(2), 173–178.

Sullivan, E. (2000). Men in nursing: The importance of gender diversity. *Journal of Professional Nursing, 16*(5), 253–254.

CHAPTER ELEVEN

Men in Nursing in Canada: Past, Present, and Future Perspectives

Wally J. Bartfay

HISTORICAL ROOTS

In Canada, the first males to provide nursing care were Jesuit mission-aries at the French garrison in Port Royal, Acadia, in 1629 (Kenton, 1925; Parkman, 1897). These men provided nursing care for the sick at a makeshift hospital in the newly founded colony (New France) and also to Aboriginal populations in the area, and were in fact the first vis-iting male nurses in Canada (Gibbon & Mathewson, 1947; Kerr, 1996). "The Jesuits singly or in pairs traveled in the depth of winter from vil-lage to village, ministering to the sick and seeking to commend their religious teachings by their efforts to relieve bodily distress" (Parkman, 1897, p. 176).

France learned about life in its new colony and the work of these first nurses in Canada over a period spanning 72 years via regular re-ports, collectively known as the *Jesuit Relations,* written by these mis-sionary priests (Kerr, 1996; Parkman, 1897). The introduction of female nursing orders in Canada occurred as a result of the cultural and societal norms of the time, which dictated that it was inappropriate for hands-on nursing care to be provided to females by male priests. For example, Father LeJeune wrote in 1634 in his *Jesuit Relations* report: "As to the men, we will take care of them according to our means; but, in regard to the women, it is not becoming for us to receive them into our houses" (Kenton, 1925, p. 49). Consequently, formal written requests were made by the Jesuit missionaries for female members of a nursing order to come to Canada to assist with their work.

The Catholic Grey Nuns (Les Soeurs Grises) of Montreal are regarded as the first female visiting nurses in Canada and were founded in 1738 by Marguerite d'Youville, who was a niece of the French explorer La Verendrye (Gibbon & Mathewson, 1947). When war broke out between England and France in 1756, the Grey Nuns opened a section of their hospital called the Ward of the English to care for wounded English soldiers (Herstein, Hughes, & Kirbyson, 1970). The transfer of authority over Montreal from the French to the British occurred in 1760.

Kerr (1996) reports that there was a marked contrast between Canada and England in the perceived status of nursing and the quality of care provided during the 17th and 18th centuries. As a consequence of King Henry VIII's renunciation of the Catholic Church in England during the 16th century (Loades, 1990), nursing orders of Catholic nuns were expelled from English hospitals and were eventually replaced by nurses of the ilk of Charles Dickens's "Sairey Gamp" (Kerr, 1996). In contrast, these negative transformations in the provision of nursing care did not occur in France or Canada to any great extent. Furthermore, the vast geographical separation from England ensured the continuation of the established French tradition of the provision of respectable nursing care in Canada by Catholic religious orders (Kerr, 1996).

PRESENT NUMBERS

Unfortunately, there is no documented statistical information on the number of male nurses practicing in Canada during the first half of the 20th century. However, in 1951, males accounted for a mere 0.33% (n = 138) of all registered nurses practicing in Canada (Canadian Nurses Association [CNA], 1960). In comparison, in 1984, 2.4% of all practicing registered nurses in Canada were male (Statistics Canada, 1985) and in 1999, 4.6% of all practicing registered nurses were male (CNA, 1999). Currently, men remain in the minority by a ratio of approximately 20 female nurses to 1 male nurse. In 2002, there were 230,957 registered nurses employed in Canada, of which 5.1% (n = 11,796) were male (Canadian Institute for Health Information, 2002). Of these male nurses, the majority practiced in the province of Quebec (44.7%), followed by 24.8% in Ontario, 10.7% in British Columbia, 6.5% in Alberta, and 4.0% in Manitoba; the remaining 9.3% were distributed through the remaining provinces and territories (Canadian Institute for Health Information, 2002).

Table 11.1 shows the percentage of male and female students enrolled in an undergraduate university degree program by province in Canada in 1996. Although 7.9% of undergraduate nursing students enrolled in university programs were male, only 4.6% (n = 10,572) of all employed registered nurses in practice were male in 1999 (CNA, 1999). These data suggest that many of the male students who began a nursing program in Canada did not complete it (Davis & Bartfay, 2001). However, it is possible that a number of practicing registered male nurses chose to leave the profession during this period.

Table 11.2 below shows the percentage of male and female students enrolled in graduate nursing degree programs in Canada by province in 1996. In total, 3.8% of these students were male. It is not clear why the percentage of male graduate nursing students is smaller than the percentage of male undergraduate nursing students. However, the absence of male nurse scholars, researchers, and theorists in university settings creates feelings of isolation and reinforces societal gender-stereotypes (Bartfay, 1996). The paucity of male role models in academia may also discourage male nurses from pursing advanced graduate training and education in nursing.

TABLE 11.1   Percentage of Male and Female Undergraduate Nursing Students Enrolled in a University Degree Program by Canadian Province

Province	% Male Students	% Female Students
Alberta	6.0	94.0
British Columbia	4.6	95.4
Manitoba	10.4	89.6
New Brunswick	8.3	91.7
Newfoundland	10.5	89.5
Nova Scotia	5.1	94.8
Ontario	7.0	93.0
Prince Edward Island	5.3	94.7
Quebec	10.0	90.0
Saskatchewan	11.7	88.2
Canada (overall)	7.9	92.1

Note: Percentages may not total 100%, due to rounding. From *University health discipline graduates*, by Statistics Canada, 1996, Ottawa, Ontario: Government of Canada.

TABLE 11.2   Percentage of Male and Female Graduate Nursing Students Enrolled in a University Degree Program by Canadian Province

Province	% Male Students	% Female Students
Alberta	1.5	98.5
British Columbia	3.0	97.0
Manitoba	5.1	94.9
New Brunswick	3.6	96.4
Newfoundland	0.0	100.0
Nova Scotia	1.9	98.1
Ontario	3.1	96.9
Prince Edward Island	0.0	0.0
Quebec	7.9	92.1
Saskatchewan	3.1	96.9
Canada (overall)	3.8	96.2

Note: Percentages may not total 100%, due to rounding. From *University health discipline graduates,* by Statistics Canada, 1996, Ottawa, Ontario: Government of Canada.

A RECENT STUDY

Methods and Sample

The aim of the study was to obtain a portrait of current Canadian attitudes and perspectives regarding men in nursing as described by male and female nursing students. Accordingly, a convenience, nonrandomized sample of current nursing students enrolled in a mid-sized comprehensive university in Ontario, Canada, was surveyed using a researcher-developed instrument. The specific research questions were as follows:

1. Do current perceptions of nursing education and practice differ between male and female nursing students enrolled in an undergraduate degree program in Ontario, Canada?
2. Do perceived barriers for recruiting and retaining men in nursing differ between male and female nursing students enrolled in an undergraduate degree program in Ontario, Canada?

This study received institutional ethical approval and conformed to Tri-Council standards for the ethical conduct of research in Canada. The study participants received an explanation and written description of the study prior to the commencement of the semester's formal lectures. The subsequent completion and return of the study's survey was regarded as informed written consent.

The items on the survey were developed by an expert panel of male and female nurses (n = 6). The items included in the survey were five Likert-type statements, to which male and female nursing students were asked to respond using the following forced-choice responses: *strongly disagree, disagree, don't know, agree or strongly agree.* These statements were as follows:

1. Overall, I believe that female nurses are superior in their *natural aptitude* for nursing.
2. Overall, I believe that female nurses are more *caring* than male nurses.
3. More efforts should be made by universities in Canada to attract increased numbers of men into the profession of nursing.
4. I feel that employers are somewhat reluctant to hire male nurses on specific units, such as women's health and obstetrics.
5. I would encourage a male family member (e.g., brother, father) to enter into the nursing profession.

The remaining items consisted of four open-ended questions, to which respondents were asked to provide their own written responses, comments, and suggestions These questions and responses are detailed in the next section. Descriptive statistics were computed for the demographic variables (e.g., age) and for the Likert-type questions. For the open-ended questions, written responses were coded and analyzed thematically.

Quantitative Findings

In all, 250 surveys were distributed and 84 were returned, resulting in a response rate of 33.6%. Of the 84 respondents, 12 (6%) were male and 72 were female. The male respondents ranged in age from 21 to 40 years, with a mean age of 24 (SD = 7). The female respondents ranged in age from 19 to 40 years, with a mean age of 23 (SD = 5). Results for the Likert-type statements are detailed in Table 11.3.

Qualitative Findings

The first open-ended question included on the survey reads as follows: "What barriers do you believe hinder more men from entering into the profession of nursing?" For the male respondents, one of the major

TABLE 11.3 Results of Likert-type Survey Items

	SA	A	DK	D	SD
"Overall, I believe that female nurses are superior in their natural aptitude for nursing."					
Male respondents	0.0%	0.0%	0.0%	33.3%	66.7%
Female respondents	0.0%	12.5%	9.7%	63.9%	13.9%
Overall	0.0%	10.7%	8.3%	59.2%	21.4%
"Overall, I believe that female nurses are more caring than male nurses."					
Male respondents	0.0%	0.0%	0.0%	58.3%	41.7%
Female respondents	0.0%	16.7%	8.3%	59.7%	15.3%
Overall	0.0%	14.2%	7.1%	59.5%	19.0%
"More efforts should be taken by universities in Canada to attract increased numbers of men into the nursing profession."					
Male respondents	25.0%	50.0%	0.0%	8.3%	16.7%
Female respondents	15.3%	33.3%	11.1%	20.8%	19.4%
Overall	16.7%	35.7%	9.5%	19.0%	19.0%
"I feel that employees are somewhat reluctant to hire male nurses on specific units such as women's health and obstetrics."					
Male respondents	0.0%	50.0%	33.3%	8.3%	8.3%
Female respondents	6.9%	44.4%	34.7%	11.1%	2.8%
Overall	6.0%	45.2%	34.5%	10.7%	3.6%
"I would encourage a male family member (e.g., brother, father) to enter into the nursing profession."					
Male respondents	33.3%	66.7%	0.0%	0.0%	0.0%
Female respondents	27.8%	50.0%	16.7%	5.6%	0.0%
Overall	28.6%	52.4%	14.3%	4.8%	0.0%

Note: SA = Strongly Agree; A = Agree ; DK = Don't Know; D = Disagree; SD = Strongly Disagree.

themes involved ridicule by family, friends, and peers. For example, one of the male respondents wrote that

> I didn't want to tell my friends in high school that I wanted to go into nursing. I know it's a good career, but society still doesn't accept males as nurses.... A lot of my high school friends still don't know b/c [because] I would be teased silly ... the butt of a thousand jokes!

A second prominent theme was the portrayal of nursing as a predominately female profession by the mass media and the entertainment industry. The following is a typical response provided by a male respondent:

> The existing stereotype [is] that it's [nursing is] for females only. Check-out TV shows and movies. Male nurses are never portrayed as hero's.... They are nurses b/c [because] they weren't good enough to go into medicine.... If you see a male nurse in the movies–TV, he's crazy, psychotic or a serial killer!!

A third theme surrounded the issue of the sexual orientation of males entering the profession. For example, one male respondent wrote: "Although I'm not gay and [I'm] happily married, a lot of people think male nurses are gay.... This has a major impact on recruitment + [and] staying."

For female respondents, a major theme involved society's labeling of men in nursing as gay and overtly feminine. For example, one female respondent wrote: "There's a social stigma that male nurses are gay or feminine. Nursing is more suited to women because of Nightingale, etc.... Many comments are made about [a] male's sexuality b/c [because] it's a caring profession. Women are generally more caring." A second theme was that nursing was not perceived by society as a manly or macho type of profession for males to pursue. The following is an example of a typical response surrounding this theme by a female respondent: "It's not [a] glamorous jock-type job like firefighters—police—being a hockey player.... There must be something wrong with them to choose this girly profession!! It's just not 'macho' to be a nurse."

The second open-ended question included on the survey read as follows: "How can schools of nursing encourage more men to apply?" A prominent theme of male respondents centered on employment opportunities and current nursing shortages in Canada. For example, one male respondent wrote that

> There's no problem for guys to get a job in nursing. Everyone knows there's a shortage of nurses in Canada.... Men are willing to take more

risks. Go to more isolated places like oil rigs, up north, travel, etc....
Women want to work in hospitals only.

Similarly, another male respondent commented that

Tell them about the economy and how you are more likely to get a job
right away. I attended a job fair last summer and 3 places want me to
work for them when I finish already. That's amazing!

A second theme was the recommendation to target men specifically in
prominent roles in strategic recruitment ads. For example, one male
respondent suggested:

There should be guys featured on nursing websites and posters.... You
can also have male nurses go into high schools to tell people that it's a
great profession with lots of vacancies. Lots of cool places to work like
ER [emergency room], med-surg [medical-surgical], or community.

Another male respondent wrote: "I found out about nursing from an
older friend who was a nurse. I got a brochure about a nursing program
with two guys on the cover, so I thought it was OK for me to apply."
A third theme involved the need for more entrance scholarships, bur-
saries, and incentives that target men specifically. One male respondent
noted:

It's pretty tough to get into university now b/c [because] it's so competitive and expensive. If you had scholarships for guys only in nursing,
I'm sure more would apply just for the money to get in.... Once they
try it, they would likely finish b/c [because] they would see how great
it is.

Similarly, another male respondent wrote: "Have scholarships dedicated
to males only.... Also have incentives for men like reduced tuition fees."
A fourth theme pertained to the word *nursing* itself as outdated and included a recommendation to change it to a more modern term. One male
respondent wrote: "Rename nursing to something else like 'Health Practitioner.' This would decrease the stigma of the word nursing.... Change
it to something males won't be as reluctant to join." A fifth theme involved specific nursing course content and nursing theory. For example,
one male respondent noted:

I'm sick and tired about reading about feminist theory. Who cares? Are
there no male researchers out there and theorists? I'm sure there are,
but feminists only want to toot their own horn.... Guys in the class

hate this bull-shit. If we say something negative or disagree, we get bad marks or fail!!

Male respondents also recommended that schools of nursing in Canada should increase the coverage of pathophysiology and basic sciences in lectures. For example, one male respondent wrote:

> There's too much touchy-feely-type stuff in nursing. Guys hate this! We want more hard stuff like interpretation of lab findings, ABGs [arterial blood gases], CBCs [complete blood count], how to read x-rays and ECGs [electrocardiograms].... No more communication stuff and holding the pt's [patient's] hand stuff.... I don't want to hear about feminist nursing theory crap anymore!!

A sixth theme was the need to increase the number of male role models and mentors in nursing. For example, one male respondent commented:

> We need to read more about males doing research and stuff. We need more male profs [professors] and clinical preceptors.... It's really a big boost for males in the class to have a male prof. [professor] teach a course like research.... We need a lot more male role models so we [males] won't leave 1/2 way through our BScN [bachelor of science in nursing].

For female respondents, a prominent theme was the need to increase the portrayal of men in nursing in the mass media and in recruitment strategies by educational and health care institutions. For example, one female respondent suggested: "Show more men on recruitment videos and posters at job fairs. This would help to show that they [males] are accepted as nurses and needed by hospitals too." Another female respondent wrote: "Have male nurses go to high schools to tell them about what nursing is today. You can also make a recruitment video with males doing stuff in various settings." A second theme involved current employment opportunities due to the shortage of nurses in Canada and the aging work force. For example, one female respondent wrote: "Advertise the need for male nurses b/c [because] of the shortage. A lot of nurses are old now, so [there are] lots of job opportunities too b/c [because] of retirements and stuff."

The third open-ended question included on the survey read as follows: "What has your experience been working with male nurses in clinical settings?" The primary theme to surface from male respondents was that male nurses were just as professional, caring, and competent as female nurses. The following provides an example of a typical response from a male respondent: "They show the same high quality care as females do.... Just as professional and dedicated." A second theme was that male nurses in practice were accepted by clients equally with their female counterparts. For example, one male respondent wrote that "They're [male nurses are] just as accepted by pt's [patients]. No problems seen so far." Another male respondent commented that "As a student it's good to see that they [male nurses] work well with female nurses, male & female MD's [medical doctors] etc. I don't think I will have any problems too."

For female respondents to the survey, the first theme to come into view was that male nurses were perceived as being just as compassionate and caring as female nurses in clinical practice. One female respondent wrote, for example: "Just as good as female nurses. I saw one cry too when their client died with the family.... Just as human and caring. No problems." The second theme to surface from female respondents was that they perceived male nurses as more interested in the technical hands-on aspects of providing care, as opposed to providing counseling to family members. For example, one female respondent wrote: "They [male nurses] are more interested in hands-on skills, i.e. dsg [dressing] changes, rather than counseling for example or psycho-social stuff." A third theme was that they perceived the male nurses in clinical settings as more powerful, influential, and assertive in nature, compared with their female counterparts. For example, one female respondent commented:

> There was this guy nurse I worked with in ortho [orthopedics] who had a lot of power & influence over the docs [doctors]. When a female nurse had problems, they would ask him to intervene and fix the problem.... He had a lot of power & influence.

The fourth open-ended question included on the survey read as follows: "What have you learned about the history of men in nursing in classes?" Surprisingly, both male and female respondents indicated that they had not been taught about the history of men in nursing and the contributions they have made. For example, one male responded: "Absolutely nothing! I think this is important to get guys motivated about nursing.... Maybe less guys would drop-out if they had some role models in history to look-up to. A *Fred Nightingale* perhaps?"

One female respondent wrote: "Zippo! I don't think men went into nursing before the 1980s— there's really no history to learn about." Interestingly, the majority of respondents said they were taught that nursing had its origins in England in the 19th century as a result of the efforts of Florence Nightingale. One male respondent noted that the "Only history we had was about Nightingale in England. She started nursing in schools—modern nursing.... nothing else learned."

Similarly, one female respondent commented: "There's a history for males??? Nothing in class. Spoke about Florence [Nightingale] and how she collected stats about death rates in hospitals and stuff.... Some stuff about Grey Nuns.... No male nurse stuff talked about in classes.

DISCUSSION

Despite the well-documented historical evidence showing that males were, in fact, the first to provide nursing care in Canada, during the early 17th century as Jesuit missionaries, male nurses are currently in the minority by a ratio of approximately 20:1. The present disproportion of males and females practicing nursing in Canada is surprising given the tremendous strides that men have made in other professions once dominated by females, including teaching, social work, and library sciences (Bartfay, 1996; Davis & Bartfay, 2001). Some of the reasons for this gender imbalance in Canada include the historical redefinition of the nurse as female by Florence Nightingale during the 19th century, gender-based societal norms, educational barriers, and legislation (Bartfay, 1996; Christman, 1988; Davis & Bartfay, 2001; Gomez, 1994; Mackintosh, 1997; Okrainec, 1990; O'Lynn, 2004).

Historically in Canada, male nurses have been blatantly discriminated against because of their gender by the Canadian armed forces (Care, Gregory, English & Venkatesh, 1996). Unlike their female counterparts in the Canadian armed forces, who were given commissions as officers with all of the associated rights and privileges, male nurses were not given similar recognition for their credentials and education until 1967. Furthermore, male nurses in the armed forces in Canada could not hold the title of nurse and were forced to be medics or orderlies. Although the number of cadets in the study sample was not formally assessed, anecdotally it is encouraging to note that both male and female officer cadets participated.

Discrimination has also been evident historically for men enrolled in nursing education programs. Even during the 20th century, with its notable social movements for equal rights and political correctness, men have been formally discriminated against by being barred from obtaining formal nursing education due to their gender (Bartfay, 1996; Davis & Bartfay, 2001; Okrainec, 1990). For example, as recently as the 1960s, only 25 out of 170 (14.7%) diploma-granting nursing schools in Canada accepted male applicants (Robson, 1964). The *official* reason for barring males from the majority of these schools was that no residential accommodations were available for them (Robson, 1964). In the province of Quebec, male nurses could not legally practice or hold the title of nurse until 1967. Hence, there was also little impetus to recruit, train, and educate male nurses in one of the most populated provinces in Canada. (Ironically, Quebec currently has the largest percentage [44.7%] of men practicing as nurses in Canada [Canadian Institute for Health Information, 2002].) Vestiges of discriminatory practices in schools of nursing may account for the high rates of attrition for male nursing students that have been reported: these are as high as 50% (Sprouse, 1996).

In light of the historical discrimination and barriers that have confronted men in nursing, it is not surprising that the results of the present survey suggest that both male and female nursing students still envision the profession of nursing from a predominately "feminine" perspective and image. The results of the present study also suggest that men face more social barriers and more of a stigma for choosing nursing as a career, in comparison to their female counterparts.

However, perspectives with regard to men in nursing may be changing. In a Canadian study of male and female students in Alberta, Okrainec (1989) reported that one-third of each group held the belief that females were superior to their male counterparts in their natural aptitude for nursing. In contrast, the results from the present study suggest that neither male nor female respondents perceive female nurses as more caring or having a superior natural aptitude for nursing.

It is interesting to note that neither male nor female respondents perceived that being male was a liability or created any barriers in terms of obtaining clinical experiences or being hired to work in specialized female units (e.g., obstetrics, women's health) upon graduation. Kerr and MacPhail (1988) report that during the 1960s and 1970s in Canada, of those nursing programs that accepted male students, many did not permit them to obtain practical clinical experience in obstetrical and gynecological hospital units. Paradoxically, male nursing students were still responsible for learning all the required obstetrical and gynecological theory covered in the curriculum, although they were not permitted to apply this theory in actual clinical practice settings. Interestingly, male *medical* students seeking practical clinical experiences in the aforementioned units did not experience these overt gender-based forms of discrimination in Canada. Okrainec (1990) reports that it was only during the 1980s that male and female nursing students finally achieved the same curriculum and clinical practice experience with clients of both sexes.

The study discussed above has some limitations. The sample represented the perspectives of one cohort of nursing students from one university program in Canada. As such, the findings may not represent the perspectives of Canadian nursing students as a whole or the perspectives of Canadian society. The perspectives of the study's nonresponders are unknown. Also, although the percentage of male participants was similar to the percentage of men in nursing in Canada, the overall number of male participants was small. In addition, the study used a cross-sectional design, prior to the completion of the students' nursing courses. However, the findings from this study differ from those of recent studies of men in nursing. From the findings of the study, a number of recommendations are offered that may continue the progress in reducing the effects of historical discrimination and barriers for men in nursing.

RECOMMENDATIONS

1. Recruitment materials prepared by universities in Canada, professional nursing associations, and health care institutions (e.g., hospitals, clinics) should make greater efforts to portray the contributions and presence of men in nursing.
2. The historical perspectives and contributions of men in nursing must be included and given equal time and treatment in nursing curricula and textbooks.
3. A consortium of university programs in Canada (e.g., the Canadian Association for Schools of Nursing) and professional nursing organizations (e.g., the Canadian Nurses Association) need to actively and aggressively lobby for the portrayal of positive male role models in the mass media and entertainment industry. Indeed, Villeneuve (1994) reports that, except for personal experience, television and the mass media are the most common sources of information about nursing for individuals of all ages.
4. University-based programs of nursing and research in Canada need to actively recruit male role models and engage in affirmative-action hiring of qualified male candidates. The lack of male nursing instructors, scholars, and researchers has profound effects on both the recruitment and the retention of males in nursing (Davis & Bartfay, 2001).
5. University programs of nursing and professional nursing organizations in Canada must support the image of nursing as a two-gender profession. As long as males remain in a minority status within nursing educational, practice, and research settings, the potential for discrimination exists, as it does for any minority group (Okrainec, 1990).
6. Local and national support groups, services, and scholarships need to be established to encourage and facilitate the recruitment and retention of men wishing either to pursue and/or to maintain a career in nursing.

REFERENCES

Bartfay, W. J. (1996). A "masculinist" historical perspective of nursing. *Canadian Nurse, 92*(2), 17–19.

Canadian Institute for Health Information. (2002). *Workforce trends of registered nurses in Canada*. Ottawa, Ontario, Canada: Author.

Canadian Nurses Association (CNA). (1960). *Facts and figures about nursing in Canada*. Ottawa, Ontario, Canada: Author.

Canadian Nurses Association (CNA). (1999). *Supply and distribution of registered nurses in Canada*. Ottawa, Ontario, Canada: Author.

Care, D., Gregory, D., English, J., & Venkatesh, P. A. (1996). A struggle for equality: Resistance to commissioning of male nurses in the Canadian military, 1952–1967. *Canadian Journal of Nursing Research, 28*(1),103–107.

Christman, L. P. (1988). Men in nursing. *Annual Review of Nursing Research, 6,* 193–205.

Davis, M. T. & Bartfay, W. J. (2001). Men in nursing: An untapped resource. *Canadian Nurse, 97*(5), 14–18.

Gibbon, J. M., & Mathewson, M. S. (1947). *Three centuries of Canadian nursing*. Toronto, Ontario, Canada: Macmillan.

Gomez, A. (1994). Men in nursing: A historical perspective. *Nurse Educator, 19*(5), 13–14.

Herstein, H. H., Hughes, L. J., & Kirbyson, R. C. (1970). *Challenge and survival: The history of Canada*. Scarborough, Ontario, Canada: Prentice-Hall of Canada.

Kenton, E. (1925). *The Jesuit relations and allied documents*. New York: The Vanguard Press.

Kerr, J. (1996). Early nursing in Canada, 1600 to 1760: A legacy for the future. In J. Kerr & J. MacPhail (Eds.), *Canadian Nursing: Issues and Perspectives* (pp. 3–10). Toronto, Ontario, Canada: Mosby.

Kerr, J., & MacPhail, J. (1988). *Canadian nursing: Issues and perspectives*. Toronto, Ontario, Canada: McGraw-Hill.

Loades, D. (1990). *Chronicles of the Tudor kings*. Wayne, NJ: CLB International.

Mackintosh, C. (1997). A historical study of men in nursing. *Journal of Advanced Nursing, 26*(2), 809–813.

Okrainec, G. (1986). Men in nursing. *The Canadian Nurse, 82*(7), 16–18.

Okrainec, G. (1989). *Perceptions of nursing education held by male and female nursing students*. Unpublished master's thesis. University of Alberta, Edmonton, Alberta, Canada.

Okrainec, G. (1990). Males in nursing: Historical perspectives and analysis. *AARN Newsletter, 46*(2), 6–8.

O'Lynn, C. E. (2004). Gender-based barriers for male students in nursing education programs: Prevalence and perceived importance. *Journal of Nursing Education, 43*(5), 229–237.

Parkman, F. (1897). *The Jesuits in North America in the seventeenth century*. Boston: Little, Brown.

Robson, R. (1964). *Sociological factors affecting recruitment into the nursing profession*. Ottawa, Ontario, Canada: Queen's Printer.

Sprouse, D. O. (1996). Message from the president. *Interaction, 14*(3), 1–4.

Statistics Canada. (1985). *Nursing in Canada: Canadian nursing statistics*. Ottawa, Ontario, Canada: Government of Canada.

Statistics Canada. (1996). *University health discipline graduates*. Ottawa, Ontario, Canada: Government of Canada.

Villeneuve, M.(1994). Recruiting and retaining men in nursing: A review of the literature. *Journal of Professional Nursing, 10*(4), 217–228.

CHAPTER TWELVE

Men in Nursing: An International Perspective

Larry D. Purnell

INTRODUCTION

There is a paucity of peer-reviewed literature on men in nursing from an international perspective. To supplement the formal literature on men in nursing from countries other than the United States and Canada, requests for information were sent to more than 50 overseas professional nursing organizations. In addition, several Listservs for nurses and nursing in the United States and overseas were accessed, requesting information on men in nursing from an international perspective. Some requests were returned because of outdated URLs; some were in languages other than the seven the author can read; others did not provide a response. Whereas many provided opinions and estimated statistics on men in nursing, few responses were thorough enough to be used in this chapter. In addition to the responses that were used, colleagues in universities and colleges in Europe, Mexico, and Asia provided anecdotal data used throughout this chapter. Thus, much of the statistical data should be viewed as relative rather than categorically imperative.

CONCEPTUAL FRAMEWORK

Because culture impacts beliefs, values, attitudes, and gender and professional roles of men and women, selected domains from the Purnell Model of Cultural Competence and the primary and secondary characteristics of culture were used to guide the development of this chapter. Space does not permit a thorough description of the model. Therefore, only a brief description is presented.

The diagram depicting the Purnell Model of Cultural Competence (see Figure 12.1) shows a circle, with an outlying rim representing global society, a second rim representing community, a third rim representing family, and an inner rim representing the person. The interior of the concentric circles is divided into 12 pie-shaped wedges depicting cultural domains and their concepts. The domains feature bidirectional arrows, indicating that each domain relates to and is affected by all other domains. Within each domain are multiple concepts. The center of the model is empty, representing unknown aspects regarding the cultural group or individual. Along the bottom of the model is a saw-toothed line representing the nonlinear concept of *cultural consciousness*. This line relates primarily to the health care provider, although organizations may also be represented on this nonlinear line according to their stage of cultural competence as organizations. The metaparadigm concepts identified in the model are *global society, community, family,* and *person* (Table 12.1). Because these metaparadigm concepts are defined from a broad perspective, they do not reflect particular national, cultural, or ethnic beliefs and values. Some languages do not have directly translatable words for these concepts. Therefore, the health care professional may need to adapt the definitions of these concepts according to the culture of the care recipient. For example, *person* may be defined differently in collectivist and individualistic cultures. In Western cultures, a person is often someone who stands alone as a unique individual. In other cultures, a person is defined in terms of the family or another group, not necessarily as a unique individual. For a more complete description of the conceptual framework, the reader is referred to the work of Purnell and Paulanka (2003).

The domains and concepts from the Purnell Model used in this chapter are (a) *overview/heritage* with the concepts economics, politics, and education, (b) *family roles and organization* with the concepts gender roles, social status, and alternative lifestyles, and (c) *workforce issues*. Table 12.2 includes a brief description of these domains and their associated concepts.

The primary characteristics of culture woven into the above domains include age, gender, and nationality. The secondary characteristics of culture woven into the above domains include educational status, socioeconomic status, political beliefs, and gender issues.

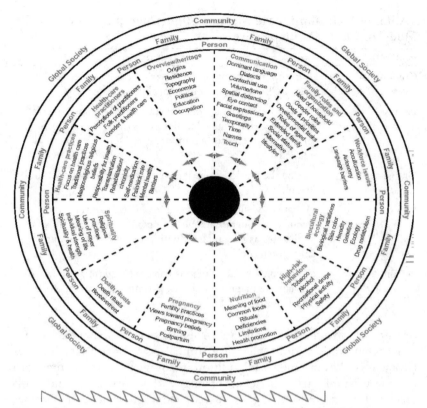

FIGURE 12.1   The Purnell Model of Cultural Competence.

OVERVIEW AND HERITAGE

Previous chapters in this book detail the early history of men in nursing. However, in the 1800 and 1900s, men were generally excluded from nursing programs, either implicitly or explicitly. After the 1950s, many countries slowly began readmitting men to nursing programs. In Czechoslovakia after 1948, the Communist government worked toward equality of men and women in the workforce (Vickers, 1999). At that time, 50% of the members of the nursing workforce were men (Fiserova, 1968). In Denmark, men entered the profession only from 1951 (Martensen, 2005) and in Sweden only from the early 1950s (Eriksson, 2002).

In Israel, very few men worked as nurses until the 1990s (Romem & Anson, 2005). However, with the shortage of nurses, Israel is now actively recruiting men into nursing with some success, although most

TABLE 12.1   Definitions of Metaparadigm Concepts of the Purnell Model of Cultural Competence

Concept	Definition
Community	A group or class of people having a common interest or identity living in a specified locality
Family	Two or more people who are emotionally involved with each other. They may, but not necessarily, live in close proximity to each other and may be blood or nonblood related
Global society	Seeing the world as one large community of multicultural people
Health	A state of wellness as defined by an ethnic or cultural group and generally including physical, mental, and spiritual states as they interact with the family, community, and global society
Person	A human being: one who is constantly adapting to his or her environment biologically, psychologically, and socially

recruits are members of minority groups from disadvantaged financial backgrounds within Israel, are from Russia, or are Israeli-Arabs (Romem & Anson, 2005). In addition, many men in Israel come into nursing with military experience, having worked as soldiers and paramedics. Few choose nursing because of parental influence but rather because they have a friend in the medical profession. Most seek nursing because of job security and promotional opportunities. Currently, over 16% of Israeli nurses are men, up from 7% 20 years ago (Romem & Anson, 2005).

Politics

China had baccalaureate nursing programs as early as 1922, although few men attended them. However, from 1952 to 1984, all higher education programs were closed under the prevailing political regime. Today, China has reopened higher education nursing programs with 5-year baccalaureate programs and a few master's programs, often with assistance from programs in the United States (Sherwood & Liu, 2005). While lecturing at four universities in Beijing, Guangzhou, and Xian, China, in 1998, the present author also visited several hospitals. No men were in any of the classes taught, nor were any men working in the intensive care units visited. However, in Hong Kong, the author interacted with several

TABLE 12.2   Selected Domains and Included Concepts from the Purnell Model of Cultural Competence

Domain	Included Concepts
Overview/Heritage	Includes concepts related to the country of origin, current residence, the effects of the topography of the country of origin and current residence, economics, politics, reasons for emigration, and value placed on education
Family Roles and Organization	Includes concepts related to the head of the household and gender roles; family roles, priorities, and developmental tasks of children and adolescents; childrearing practices and roles of the aged and extended family members; individual and family social status in the community; and views toward alternative lifestyles such as single parenting, sexual orientation, childless marriages, and divorce
Workforce Issues	Includes concepts related to autonomy, acculturation, assimilation, gender roles, ethnic communication styles, and health care practices from the country of origin

men in nursing, most of whom were in academia and had been educated in Great Britain. The Shanghai Board of Nursing (2005) reports that 7.8% of its nurses are men. Whether or not this number is representative of the country as a whole is unknown.

In Portugal, men have been an integral part of the nursing profession since the dictatorship government in the middle of the 20th century. If men went into nursing, they did not have to enlist in the military (Antonio Carlos, personal communication, May 2004). Because men were recognized as being integral to the profession, today 22.9% of nurses are men (Orden dos Enfermerios, 2005). While giving a presentation at an international conference and touring nursing classrooms at the University of Beja in Beja, Portugal, in 2004, it appeared to the present author that the audience at the conference was at least 40% male, with nursing classes approaching 35–40% men.

Education and Socioeconomic Status

In the European Union, women on the average make 79% of what men make in the same occupational category, with the percentage of difference ranging from 88% in Sweden to 67% in Portugal and 70% in Greece and the Netherlands (International Council of Nurses, 2003b). Men in nursing attain the types of further training and specialization likely to lead to promotion and better pay. In Great Britain, where 9.4% of nurses are men, men hold 45% of academic and senior management positions. However, among higher positions, there is no salary difference by gender or ethnicity (International Council of Nurses, 2003b; Royal College of Nursing and Midwifery Council, 2002). One of the reasons given for the imbalance is that 64% of women but only 28% of men take some form of career break.

However, in Czechoslovakia during the 1970s and 1980s, women attained higher educational levels than did men and were more likely than men to become scientists, white-collar professionals, and medical personnel (Bitusikova, 2003). Consequently, the percentage of men in nursing was higher (at times up to 50%) than in other European countries.

In Saudi Arabia, the Ministry of Health is attempting to support men in nursing (Samarkandi, 2005). A number of nursing schools in the United States have set up programs for Saudi Arabian men, one of the most notable being at George Mason University in Fairfax, Virginia (George Mason University, 2001).

FAMILY ROLES AND ORGANIZATION

Culture is primarily learned and passed on in the family. Men and women learn from an early age, based in the family context, the gender roles and behavior that are acceptable. Additionally, they learn which occupations and professions are acceptable for men and for women, as well as which are accorded high status and respect. Society's perception of certain behaviors as masculine or feminine has a powerful influence on young adults considering a career.

Gender and Gender Issues

With only one exception, judging by what could be found in the professional and lay literature, nurses worldwide are overwhelmingly female. The one exception is in Francophone Africa (Benin, Burkino Faso, Cameroon, Chad, Congo, Côte d'Ivoire, the Democratic Republic of Congo, Djibouti, Guinea, Gabon, Mali, Mauritania, Niger, Rwanda, Senegal, and Togo) where more men than women are nurses (*Francophone Africa*, 2004). However, midwives are entirely female in Africa (International Council of Nurses, 2003a). Only about 1% of nurses in Iceland are men (Kristinsson, 2001), while over 20% of nurses are men in Spain (M. Lillo Crespo, personal communication, June 2004), Portugal (Orden dos Enfermerios, 2005), Czechoslovakia (Bitusikova, 2003), and Italy (Kristinsson, 2001) (see appendix to this chapter).

Professional and lay literature from every country from which information on men in nursing could be retrieved portray nursing as a predominantly female profession or occupation requiring stereotyped feminine traits such as caring, nurturing, submissiveness, dependence, emotional expressiveness, and attentiveness to detail in contrast to perceived masculine traits such as dominance, strength, aggression, leadership, technical knowledge, and dedication. Whereas views on these traits seem to be changing, especially within nursing, the public still holds these stereotypical views about femininity and masculinity. Consequently, many men are reluctant to enter the profession, and some do not even consider it as an option.

Traditional views of men have been changing to new views of men in many countries, starting with the gender equality movements in Sweden in the late 1960s and early 1970s. The traditional perspective was problematic for men seeking role models in nursing (Nolberg, 2004). Although the new man is considered to be pleasant and emotional, he must still look like a so-called real man. Currently, this view is moderated by simply viewing men as having a different perspective from women. Because the word for nurse in Sweden is a feminine word, *sjuksköterskao,* some believe that this continues to deter men from entering the profession (Vaxjo University, 2005), even though men have been entering nursing in Sweden since the early 1950s (Eriksson, 2002).

Alternative Lifestyles

Another theme that appears repeatedly in the literature is a perception that men in nursing are gay. According to Fisher and Connell (2000), who echo much of the international perspective, male nurses generally believe that one of the major reasons why men do not go into nursing is that the public may assume they are gay. To combat this stereotype, some heterosexual men in nursing employ homophobic behaviors (Fisher & Connell, 2000). Another way in which male nurses decrease this stigmatization is to practice in areas that are perceived as high tech and more masculine, such as anesthesiology, intensive care/critical care, and emergency/shock trauma (Armstrong, 2002; Fisher & Connell, 2000). In addition, these areas frequently attract higher prestige and higher pay. Of course, these perceptions are based on patriarchal ideas of masculinity.

Interestingly, recent research suggests that men have as many female attributes as women have. Therefore, men are just as suited for nursing as women (Fisher, 1999). For men to be successful in nursing where women dominate the profession, some believe they must adapt to the feminine nature of the profession (Watson, 1999). However, others believe that as technology in nursing takes on a more important role, the profession will be seen as more masculine and, therefore, nursing will be of more interest to men (Watson, 1999).

Social Status

Because nursing historically has been perceived as subordinate to many other professions, the social status of nursing appears to be an issue for men entering nursing. Social status is usually determined by economics and education. As nursing gains a more professional image and as salary equity between men and women becomes realized, more men, it appears, go into nursing (Mackintosh, 1997).

Spanish men have been highly visible in nursing leadership roles, a fact that is possibly related to the value Spanish society has historically attributed to men. If you look at Spanish celebrations, festivals, customs, and traditions, differences between men's and women's roles are clear. Men's roles are usually related to power and strength, while women's roles are passive. Though Spanish society is not supposed to be so *machista* today, these attitudes are still both implicit and explicit in everyday life. Men get better professional positions, and political issues are dealt with mostly by men. In this context, even though more women than men are nurses in Spain, the profession is dominated by men who occupy executive positions, policymaking positions, and research and academic positions in nursing (Lillo Crespo, 2002).

Historically, in Spain, men have enjoyed better educational opportunities and have advanced into specialized roles. In fact, in the past there were different educational levels inside nursing, with men holding the top positions. In the first 60 years of the 20th century, male nurses were called *practicantes:* these represented the highest level of nursing. Their fame came from their preparation as technicians. They were considered nearly equivalent to physicians and achieved powerful positions, especially in small villages and towns where physicians were many miles distant. On the other hand, female nurses were informal caregivers or servants and their education, including that of midwives, was lower: in some cases, their training did not include formal education (Lillo Crespo, 2002). Although women are making progress in Spain, many female nurses are not yet ready to sacrifice their personal lives to establish equality with men (Lillo Crespo, 2002). Other countries in Southern Europe may be in the same situation as Spain due to their strong core values related to men, autonomy, and power (Melkas, 2004; Nolberg, 2004; *This Is Norway*, 2002).

Northern European countries have historically developed societies in which men and women are equally respected and have the same opportunities. In these countries, the principles of justice and equality are crucial to make their societies work. A Spanish student makes this observation:

> My last year as a nursing student, I stayed in Norway with a grant from my university. I could appreciate that everybody had the same chance as a professional in every area. Women have had a high specific weight in their society and even their laws and moral issues are focused mostly on women needs. Countries in Central Europe have conserved a very classic image of the nursing profession and that's why the number of men nurses is very small. Besides these countries have not had a big development of nursing from the education and the clinical practice perspective. Maybe the lack of leadership in their nurses has been the cause why not a lot of men have been attracted by this profession. (quotation supplied by M. Lillo Crespo, personal communication, April 20, 2005)

When a man in nursing belongs to one of the racial groups that have lower social status and limited opportunities in some societies, he may suffer a double stigma, stigmatizing both his masculinity/sexuality and also his race (*Male Nursing Forum*, 2005). In Israel, Israeli Arabs continue to face discrimination in hiring practices (Romem & Anson, 2005).

To achieve the societal recognition of nursing and to increase the status of nurses in South Korea, Mo Im Kim, the first Asian president of the International Council of Nurses, campaigned to change the language referring to a nurse. Originally, the Korean word for nurse was *kanhobu*, the ending *bu* connoting *housewife*. After 1945, the Korean word for nurse was changed to *kanhowon*, with the ending *won* connoting *worker*. Finally in 1987, the word for nurse was changed to *kanhosa*, with the ending *sa* connoting *teacher*. In the highly honorific Korean language, words referring to professionals end with *sa*, as in *uisa* for doctor, *pyonhsa* for lawyer, and *yaksa* for pharmacist. Changing the name given to nurses gives them a better self-image, and nurses are elevated in the public's recognition of them (Cho & Kashka, 1998; Kim, 1998). Increasing the status of the nursing profession, it is suggested, also means that more men will seek nursing as a career. In the 1970s, only 3% of nurses in Korea were men. Currently, it is estimated that 12% of nurses are men, an increase of 9% over a 20-year period (Chung Nam Kim, personal communication, October 2002). However, it is not known if the increase in men in nursing is due to other changes in Korean society. In addition, nurses in Korea raise their status and increase their opportunities to obtain grants and positions if they publish in a U.S.-based journal (Choo, 2005).

The low status of nursing as a profession, not to be misinterpreted as a lack of respect for nurses, in many countries has been attributed to the fact that nursing has been dominated by females who are culturally expected to practice in a physician-dominated system such as the system in Nicaragua (Zamora, 1998), the system in Pakistan, where the status of nurses is exacerbated by the low status of women in a Muslim society (Jan, 1996), and the system in patriarchal Japan (Anders & Kanai-Pak, 1992). In Arab Middle-Eastern countries, where educated people prefer white-collar jobs and nursing is seen as menial labor, few men go into nursing (Kulwicki, 2003). In Sweden, nursing has not been seen as a desirable profession and has not been encouraged among males from childhood, because nursing has suffered from a low status and low wages, and it is seen as women's work (Eriksson, 2002).

In Iceland, the view of nursing is that the work of nursing is monotonous and requires little education and that men who go into nursing are different from other men and lose their masculinity (Blondal, 2004; WENR, 2001). Thus, the few men who do go into nursing (less than one percent) go into emergency, intensive care, psychiatric, operating room, or anesthesia nursing or they go to other countries where prejudices about men in nursing are less apparent (WENR, 2001). To combat this perception of men in nursing, the University of Iceland initiated a campaign to attract men to nursing and was successful in enrolling 22 men in its freshman class in the year 2000. However, at the end of the first year, only one male student remained in the class (Kristinsson, 2001). As in so many other places in the world, it seems easier to attract men into the nursing profession; but retaining them in school and into the workforce is more difficult.

Despite the low status that nursing may present to men, some believe that if more men are attracted to nursing, the status of the profession will increase, but that this will also put more pressure on men to "rescue nursing" (Evans, 2004). According to Waters, Postic, Durocher, Donker et al. (1999), at least in some segments of the international community, an increased number of men in nursing has given greater prestige and status to nursing, primarily due to the increased education, motivation, and assertiveness of both male and female nurses.

WORKFORCE ISSUES

A study in Germany reported that younger men in nursing had a higher tendency to leave nursing than did women or older men, especially among those working in hospitals. In addition, the desire to leave the profession was more pronounced among nurses with a specialization (Hasselhorn et al., 2004). The reason for men leaving nursing at higher rates than women was not determined, but burnout was the most frequent reason for leaving nursing among all the study's participants. However, some possible reasons for men leaving might include poor salary progression beyond the entry level salary, a phenomenon common throughout the nursing profession in many countries (International Council of Nurses, 2003a).

As in Germany, men in nursing in Great Britain are generally less satisfied with nursing as a career than women are. Minority men are even less satisfied, believing that they are harassed and lack opportunities to progress. In addition, men are more likely to work in mental health, learning disabilities, and adult critical care than are women and tend to enter the profession at a later age than do women, age 26 for men versus age 23 for women (Royal College of Nursing and Midwifery Council, 2002).

RECOMMENDATIONS

The current shortage of nurses is a global phenomenon. In order to meet the world's nursing and health care needs, nursing must recruit men and other underrepresented groups into the profession. The barriers to admitting men or any other group into the profession must be removed. The following are some recommendations designed to increase the number of male nurses. Some of these recommendations are more appropriate to some countries than to others:

- Professional nursing organizations must work to decrease any stigma with regard to men entering nursing. Nursing organizations should abolish the oppressive sex-role differentiation reflected in current conditions and upbringings and social expectations.
- Men should join women's groups, which have made great strides in some countries toward gender and employment equality. Gender equality will not occur until the external image of nursing is changed in the eyes of the public.
- Nurses should speak well of nursing. If pride is not taken in the profession, then others will not see the profession as desirable.

- Nurses and their organizations should seize every opportunity to include pictures of men in nursing in print and live media.
- Colleges and universities and health care employers must recruit men in elementary and high schools, at sporting events, in churches, and in public places where young men congregate.
- Nursing organizations should encourage community newspapers to publish stories of men in nursing.
- Nursing organizations should use strategies specific to the ethnicity of the population being recruited.
- Nursing schools and colleges should make guidance counselors aware of the opportunities for men in nursing.
- Nursing schools and colleges should post signs in public transportation facilities, encouraging men in nursing.
- Nursing schools and colleges should recruit men at community days, county fairs, summer camps, and in the military at ROTC venues.
- Nursing organizations should encourage men interested in a second career to consider nursing.
- Nursing schools and colleges should increase the number of weekend, evening, and online nursing programs.
- Nursing organizations should encourage mentoring programs in nursing. Recruiting men into the profession is only part of the supply concern. Once in school or in the profession, institutions should make every effort to achieve retention.
- Colleges, universities, and health care employers should educate the public about men in nursing.

CONCLUSION AND COMMONALITIES

Nursing, as a global phenomenon, continues to be a profession dominated by females in most of the world, the one exception being in Francophone Africa. The underlying reasons why men do not go into nursing are multifactoral and include the perception of men in nursing being gay: perhaps this is more of a concern for some than for others. The main international commonality in terms of why men go into nursing is socioeconomics: they will have job security. Currently, most men seek nursing positions in critical care areas, psychiatric and disability settings, the military, and administration. As salaries in the nursing profession increase, men may see the nursing profession as more viable.

Most Western societies assume, stereotypically, that men are not as caring as women when it comes to nursing. In this regard, men in nursing are good role models for children and for other men and women. In conclusion, if each country could increase men in nursing by just a modest 1% to 2% a year, impressive numbers could be reached within a decade.

REFERENCES

Anders, R., & Kanai-Pak, M. (1992). Death from overwork: A nursing problem in Japan? *Nursing & Health Care, 13*(4), 187–192.

Armstrong, F. (2002). Not just women's business: Men in nursing. [Electronic version]. *Australia Nursing Journal, 9*(11), 24–26. Retrieved January 2, 2005, from http://www.findarticles.com/p/articles/mi_go2126/is_200206/ai_n7059498

Bitusikova, A. (2003). *Women's social entitlements in Slovakia.* Paper presented at the Network for European Women Rights Conference, Athens, Greece, October 10–11, 2003. Retrieved March 24, 2005, from http://www.newr.bham.ac.ud/pdfs/Social?Slovakia%20report.pdf

Blondal, L. (2004, November). *Changes in Icelandic organizational structure.* Paper presented at the conference on the Nordic Labor Market, Reykjavik, Iceland.

Charles Sturt University. (2005). *Student news.* Retrieved March 25, 2005, from http://www.csu.edu.au/division/marketing/billboard/1213/student.htm

Cho, H., & Kashka, M. (1998). Change in the word symbol for nurse in Korea. *Image: Journal of Nursing Scholarship, 30*(3), 265–268.

Choo, J. (2005, Winter). Connected to the world through scholarship: Visiting scholars. *The Pitt Nurse,* 22–23.

Eriksson, H. (2002). *Den diplomatiska punkten—Maskulinitet som kroppsligt identitetsskapande project i svensk sjukskoterskeutbilnning* [The Diplomatic Point—Masculinity as an embodied identity project in Swedish nursing education]. Göteborg, Sweden: Acta Universitatis Gothoburegensis.

Evans, J. (2004) Men nurses: A historical and feminist perspective. *Journal of Advanced Nursing, 47*(3), 321–328.

Fiserova, J. (1968). Job satisfaction of hospital physicians and nurses. *Czeck Zdrow, 3*(16), 126–151.

Fisher, M. (1999). Sex role characteristics of men in nursing. *Contemporary Nurse, 8*(5), 65–71.

Fisher, M., & Connell, R. (2000). *Masculinities and men in nursing.* Retrieved March 20, 2005, from www.chs.usyd.edu.au/conf2002/minipost/gx-fishe.pdf

Francophone Africa. (2004). Retrieved April 17, 2005, from the University of Portsmouth, England, Web site: http://www.hum.port.ac.uk/slas/francophone/country.htm

George Mason University. (2001). *George Mason University offers education to Saudi Arabian students.* Retrieved April 20, 2005, from http://www.gmu.edu/news/release/saudiarabia.html

Hasselhorn, H., Tackenberg, P., Buscher, A., Stelzig, S., Kummerling. A., & Muller, B. (2003). *Intent to leave nursing in Germany.* Retrieved March 15, 2005, from http://www.next.uni-wuppertal.de/download/Buch2003/ch15.pdf

Hiranprueck, A. (2004). *Thailand nurse workforce factsheet.* Retrieved April 2, 2005, from http://66.102.7.104/search?q = cache:ouyj5WBZwvYJ:www.nursing.virginia.edu/centers/srmhrc/ThailandNurseWorkforceFactSheet_final.doc+Thailand+workforce+fact+sheet&hl = en

Instituto Nacional de Estadistica, Mexico [National Institute of Statistics, Mexico]. (2004). Retrieved April 19, 2004, from http://www.inegi.gob.mx/inegi/contenidos/espanol/prensa/contenidos/estadisticas/2004/enfermera04.pdf

International Council of Nurses. (2003a). *ICN Workforce Forum Report.* Retrieved April 4, 2005, from www.icn.ch/forum2003report.pdf

International Council of Nurses. (2003b). *Nursing matters: ICN fact sheet [Equal opportunities: Gender issues].* Retrieved January 2, 2005, from http://www.icn/ch/matter_equalop.htm

Jan, R. (1996). A cultural dilemma: Pakistani nursing. *Reflections, 22*(4),1 9.

Kim, M. (1998). Breaking traditions: A personal reflection. *Reflections, 24*(4), 14–17.

Kristinsson, P. (2001). Fields of masculinity: Icelandic men in nursing. Retrieved February 10, 2005, from http://aukavefir.hjukrun.is/veistu/

Kulwicki, A. (2003). People of Arab ancestry. In L. Purnell & B. Paulanka (Eds.), *Transcultural health care: A culturally competent approach* (2nd ed., pp. 90–106). Philadelphia: F. A. Davis.

Lillo Crespo, M. (2002). Antropologia, genero y enfermeria contemporanea [Anthropology, gender, and contemporary nursing]. *Revista ROL de Enfermeria, 25*(12), 56–62.

Mackintosh, C. (1997). A historical study of men in nursing. *Journal of Advanced Nursing, 2*(26), 232–236.

Male Nursing Forum. (2005). Retrieved March 12, 2005 from http://allnurses.com

Martensen, S. (2005). *Guestbook men in nursing.* Retrieved March 13, 2005, from http://www.geocities/Athens/Forum/6011/geobook.html

Melkas, H. (2004, November). *Gender segregation in Nordic labour markets: Trends and challenges.* Paper presented at the conference on the Nordic Labour Market, Reykjavik, Iceland.

Nolberg, M. (2004, November). *Gender flexible models for gender transformation or for hegemonic masculinity?* Paper presented at the conference on the Nordic Labor Market, Reykjavik, Iceland.

Orden dos Enfermerios [National Registration Board—Portugal]. (2005). Author.

Purnell, L., & Paulanka, B. (2003). *Transcultural health care: A culturally competent approach.* Philadelphia: F. A. Davis.

Romem, P., & Anson, O. (2005). Israeli men in nursing: Social and personal motives. *Journal of Nursing Management, 13*(2), 173–178.

Royal College of Nursing and Midwifery Council. (2002). *Valued equally?* Retrieved March 26, 2005, from http://www.rcn.org.uk/publications/pdf/survey-2002

Samarkandi, O. (2005, Winter). Student snapshot. *Pitt Nurse,* 19.

Shanghai Nursing Board. (2005). Retrieved April 2, 2005, from http://www.snb.gov.sg/

Sherwood, G., & Liu, Huaping, L. (2005). International collaboration for developing graduate education in China. *Nursing Outlook, 53,* 15–20.

This Is Norway: Women at work. (2002). Retrieved January 2, 2005, from http://www.ssb.no/norge_en/arbeid_en

Vaxjo University. (2005). Retrieved January 2, 2005, from http://www/vxu.se//avhandlingar/sune_dufwa.html

Vickers, E. (1999). Frances Elisabeth Crowell and the politics of nursing in Czechoslovakia after the first world war. *Nursing History Review, 7,* 67–96.

Waters, K., Postic, M., Durocher, S., Donker, H., & Benenr, B. (1999). Janforum. *Journal of Advanced Nursing, 29*(2), 523.

Watson, J. (1999). *Postmodern nursing and beyond.* London: Churchill Livingstone.

WENR (Workgroup of European Nurse Researchers). (2001). Retrieved January 2, 2005 from http://www/wenr.org/view_categories.phb?nCatID = 34

Zamora, L. (1998). Equity's powerful hold on dreams. *Reflections, 24*(2), 12–13.

Percentage of Men in Nursing by Country*

Country	% Nurses as Men	Comments
Australia	9%	Charles Sturt University reports that 50% of the students enrolled in one nursing class in 2003.
China	7.8%	These figures are specific to Shanghai and may not be representative of the rest of China. (S. Lu, personal communication, April 5, 2005.)
Czech Republic	10–50%	In previous decades, most physicians started as nurses in Slovakia. These percentages depend on how men nurses are counted.
Denmark	3.5%	The first men in nursing were in 1951.
England	10%	Percentage has been slowly, but steadily, increasing from 8.87% in 1994. Men more commonly work in mental health, disabilities, critical care or administration. On the average, men enter the profession three years later than do women. Men take advantage of opportunities for higher education and accept senior/management positions at a higher rate than do women.
Finland	7%	
Francophone Africa	50+%	
Hungary	9.7%	In 2000, the percentage of nurses who were men was 8%. (J. Betlehem, personal communication, March 20, 2005.)

(Continued)

Country	% Nurses as Men	Comments
Israel	16.5%	Most are Israeli-Arabs or Russians who emigrated from the USSR after 1989.
Italy	20%	
Korea	12%	The number of men has been increasing after the word symbol for nurse was changed, making it professional and gender neutral. Nurses who get academic education in the USA and who publish in an American journal have higher status then those who publish in a Korean journal.
Mexico	9.5%	In group meetings in Mexico with nurses who express interest in migrating to the USA, men represented about 15% of the audience.
New Zealand	7.7%	No evidence was found for active efforts to recruit
Nicaragua	2%	Nursing is perceived as women's work. (C. Ross, personal communication, March 25, 2005.)
Norway	10%	?
Panama	8%	There are only BSN programs, with 2000+ applicants for 100 positions each year at the University of Panama.
Philippines	25%	Some men go into nursing as a means to have a profession for emigration.
Portugal	22.9%	Before 1974, if men became nurses, they did not have to join the military.
Saudi Arabia	?	Most nurses working in Saudi Arabia come from Lebanon or Jordan. The Ministry of Health is encouraging men to enter the nursing profession. (Z. Fedorowicz, personal communication, March 25, 2005.)
Scotland	10%	

Country	% Nurses as Men	Comments
Spain	20+%	In decades past, men worked as practicantes who were considered the highest ranked among nurses, especially in rural areas.
		Practicantes functioned similarly as physician's assistants in the USA.
		Men tend to go into specialties and attain more education than do women. Nursing is currently dominated by men.
Sweden	7%	One reason given for the low numbers of men in nursing is that the word for nurse in Swedish is a feminine-marked word. Sweden is currently using the Johnson & Johnson film to recruit men into nursing.
Thailand	10%	Men comprise 7.6% of nursing faculty positions. Technical nurses must obtain a BSN by 2006.
Wales	8%	

* Statistics of men in nursing vary greatly according to who reports them. The figures provided in this table are from government Web sites, professional organizations, or the most knowledgeable sources available and are listed here or in the references for this chapter.

PART IV

Future Directions

Nursing has a rich and proud heritage. Nursing has faced wars, pestilence, and change with grace. The future of nursing looms large with profound issues. Genome research indicates a new and different way of treating illness, and the practice of medicine will truly be radically altered. A spill-over into nursing is guaranteed. Nursing also faces a significant challenge in the increasing demand for nursing care by an aging population when its most educated teachers and leaders are themselves aging.

One solution to the problem of increasing the supply of nurses requires a change in traditional recruitment methods to attract ethnic and gender minorities. Diversity in nursing consists of educational programs rather than ethnic and gender balance. The chapters in part IV explore recruitment and retention barriers for men in nursing and offer suggestions as to how the desired goals may be achieved. Just as in fishing you have to use the correct bait to catch the desired fish, in recruiting nontraditional groups to nursing you have to change your methods. Nursing's future requires change, and part IV points out the possibilities.

— Russell E. Tranbarger

CHAPTER THIRTEEN

Recruitment and Retention of Men in Nursing

Susan A. LaRocco

INTRODUCTION

In 2000, there were almost 2.7 million registered nurses (RNs) with active licenses in the United States: approximately 2.55 million women and 146,902 men, representing 5.4% of the total RN population (Spratley, Johnson, Sochalski, Fritz, and Spencer, 2001). More than 2.2 million RNs (82% of the total) are currently employed in nursing, of whom approximately 129,000 are male, accounting for 5.9% of all RNs employed in nursing. Buerhaus, Staiger, and Auerbach (2004), using data from the Current Population Study, report that the percentage of men in the nursing workforce had increased to slightly more than 8.5% in 2003. Using this same data source, Buerhaus et al. estimate that the percentage of men in the nursing workforce in 2000 was approximately 7.5%. Whether the most accurate figure for the percentage of men in the nursing workforce is approximately 6% or almost 9% is, for the most part, irrelevant. Either estimate indicates that men are woefully underrepresented in the nursing workforce.

Although the percentage of men in the nursing workforce in other countries varies significantly, underrepresentation of men in nursing is an international phenomenon. In Canada, just over 5% of all nurses are male, with almost half practicing in Quebec, a province that did not even license men as nurses until 1969 (Canadian Nurses Association, 2003). In Ireland, men now account for approximately 8% of all nurses in the workforce, while in the United Kingdom, 10% of all nurses are men (International Council of Nurses, 2004). In Germany, men comprise 18% of the nursing workforce (German Nurses Association, 2004).

The underrepresentation of men in nursing has historical roots. Despite relatively recent calls to increase the number of men in nursing, barriers to the effective recruitment and retention of men in nursing persist. This chapter will review the origins of these barriers and discuss the findings of two recent studies in which men nurses provide their perspectives on strategies that might break down the barriers.

HISTORICAL PERSPECTIVE

Although men have been functioning as nurses since ancient times, their exclusion from nursing and discrimination against them has been common since the Nightingale era. Nightingale succeeded in creating a respectable occupation for women, as it was considered natural in Victorian England for nursing care to be provided by women. Nightingale believed that men were not fit to be nurses but that "every woman is a nurse" (1860, p. 3). The establishment of nurses' homes, where all nursing students resided, was also instrumental in preventing men from being considered for admission to the newly established training schools structured after Nightingale's model for schools of nursing. Building separate residences for men was not considered, as there was no desire or perceived need to accommodate male nursing students.

In the United States, there has also been a long history of discrimination against men in nursing. The Army Nurse Corps, Female, was established in 1901. Male nurses were barred from serving as nurses in the military until 1955 (Bullough, 1997). Men were also barred from the American Nurses Association until a membership bylaws revision in 1930 finally allowed properly qualified male nurses to join that organization (Bullough, 2001).

IS GENDER DIVERSITY IMPORTANT?

In terms of gender, authors have discussed whether gender diversity in nursing is beneficial to the profession as a whole, to nurses' clients, and to the individual man who either is a nurse or aspires to become a nurse. Sullivan (2000), in an editorial strongly supporting the need for gender diversity in nursing, notes that nursing administrators support the concept that "the profession must reflect a variety of ethnic, racial, cultural, and religious background to provide care to the wide [and growing] diversity of our patients" (p. 253). She contends that although gender diversity is essential, it is seldom addressed by administrators. Sullivan states that "Anything other than full equality for men in nursing is nothing less than shameful" (p. 254).

Christman (1974), a male nurse and international nurse leader who experienced discrimination in many arenas, describes many female nurses as having a "start-stop" career pattern, withdrawing from the workforce with the birth of each child. He argues that having a larger percentage of men in nursing would produce a more stable workforce and would reduce the shortage of nurses. He indicates that there was an artificial shortage of nurses in the early 1970s because many licensed nurses were not working in nursing during their child-rearing years. While his argument may seem somewhat dated, because nowadays more women stay in the workforce while raising children, it remains true today that women are more likely to take time off from work around the birth of a child than are men.

Others are less enthusiastic about gender diversity in nursing. Ryan and Porter (1993) argue against the importance of gender diversity in nursing. Ryan and Porter review the British experience with an increased number of men in nursing and conclude that having more men in nursing in the United States would not improve the occupation's professional status. They base their argument on the belief that there are two problems associated with an increased number of men in nursing. The first is the tendency for men in nursing to advance to administrative positions, thus gaining a disproportionate voice in professional organizations, resulting in dominance over female nurses. The second problem is that there is no guarantee that an increased number of men in nursing will improve the status of nursing among other health professions. Ryan and Porter conclude that "In light of the U.K. experience ... it would be more profitable for American nurses to put their energies into building on feminist strategies, rather than placing their trust in men to be the saviors of the occupation" (p. 267).

Likewise, London (1987) cautions against the recruitment of men into nursing. London examined the impact of an increased number of men in education careers in the United States and the increased number of men in nursing careers in Great Britain. In both cases, she found that men tended to dominate the administrative positions, which resulted in more masculine control of the professions. She concludes that "If men dominated the leadership, the oppressed group behavior currently keeping nursing in its submissive place would be internally reinforced" (p. 79). She views nursing "as an intrinsically female profession, based on female values and morals and a holistic world view" (p. 80).

In the current era, which places an emphasis on political correctness, it would not be popular to advocate that men be excluded from nursing.

Indeed, in many places significant efforts are being made to actively recruit men into nursing. While these efforts may reflect a truly egalitarian spirit, it is also likely that they represent a need to increase the overall number of nurses in order to prevent a critical shortage. In response to media coverage of a looming nursing shortage, schools of nursing have seen an increased number of enrollment applications from many more qualified applicants than can be accommodated (American Association of Colleges of Nursing, 2005b). As nursing schools fill to capacity with students, it is possible that recruitment efforts aimed at increasing the number of men in nursing may become less widespread. However, decreasing the recruitment efforts targeting men will not improve the overall gender diversity in nursing.

BARRIERS TO RECRUITMENT

Several issues have been cited as barriers to recruiting men into nursing. These include low salaries (Barkley & Kohler, 1992; Gorman, 2003; Halloran & Welton, 1994; Poliafico, 1998; Villeneuve, 1994), the traditionally feminine image of nursing (Evans, 1997; MacPhail, 1996; Okrainec, 1994; Poliafico, 1998), the image of men nurses as homosexuals (Boughn, 1994; Gray et al., 1996; Mangan, 1994; Rallis, 1990; C. L. Williams, 1995), the lack of status in nursing (Kelly, Shoemaker, & Steele, 1996; C. L. Williams, 1992), a lack of awareness regarding the opportunities in nursing (Boughn, 1994; Bullough, 1994; Kelly, Shoemaker, & Steele, 1996), and even the word nurse itself (Gorman, 2003; Villeneuve, 1994).

Salaries for full time RNs employed in nursing rose from $46,782 to $57,784 between 2000 and 2004. This represents a 12.4% increase in real earnings as adjusted for consideration of inflation (Health Resources and Services Administration, 2004). However, the public perception that wages are low remains a barrier for men. In a survey of 100 male suburban high-school juniors, Gorman (2003) found that the students had a generally favorable impression of nursing as a career for men; however, they didn't think that nursing paid very well. This finding is interesting since in the geographic area where the survey was conducted, new graduate nurses were obtaining starting salaries in excess of $50,000 and it was not uncommon for experienced nurses to earn more than $100,000 (Donna Jenkins, personal communication, 2005).

The traditionally feminine image of nursing includes the common stereotypes of nurses, such as the ministering angel, the battle-ax, the sex symbol, and the doctor's handmaiden. None of these images are likely to appeal to men or boys exploring career options. While these images have little bearing on current reality, their perpetuation in the media likely makes it difficult for a young man to see himself as a nurse. In addition, the feminine language often used to refer to nursing and the feminine colors and images used in nursing-school literature present an obstacle to overcome when a man considers nursing. Other practices, such as commandeering the men's room for use by women attendees at nursing conventions, reinforce the image of nursing as a strictly female profession.

The perception that many or most men who are nurses are effeminate or homosexual may also deter some men from considering nursing. Bush (1976) reports that one-third of the male nurses in her study were asked at some point if they were gay. Rallis (1990), in a small informal survey, reports that the men he interviewed strongly disapproved of male nurses and "most assumed that all male nurses are gay" (p. 160). Kelly et al. (1996) report that male nursing students described fear of being considered unmanly and some reported that they felt a need to mention their wife or children or to prominently display a wedding band in order to display their heterosexuality.

Traditionally female-dominated professions are considered by society to be of lower status than occupations that attract mostly men (C. L. Williams, 1992). Kelly et al. (1996) report that male nursing students said the public image of nursing was negative. Students described the public perception of nursing as "mundane, subservient, an occupation rather than a profession" (p. 171). For the students, men who took a traditionally female position would be considered as taking a step down the social ladder.

Since words often carry strong associations, periodically the question is raised as to whether the word nurse is a deterrent for some men with regard to choosing the profession. Gorman (2003) found in his study of 100 male high-school students that only six indicated an interest when asked if they would consider a career as a nurse; this number changed to 21 when he renamed the profession with the gender-neutral title of registered clinician.

EARLY EFFORTS TO RECRUIT MEN

Recruitment strategies to increase the number of men in nursing in Britain began as early as 1943. The Ministry of Health provided condensed courses for ex-servicemen in 1943 and again in 1949 and developed literature that would encourage men to consider nursing as a career (Mackintosh, 1997). In Canada, the Ontario Hospital Association began a campaign to increase the number of men in nursing in

1967. They developed a pamphlet titled *There Is a Place for Men in the Nursing World* (Evans, 2004) which was distributed to high-school boys. In the United States, a program called Med-Vet, which was supported by a federal grant, was developed at a community college in Texas to provide medical corpsmen (male and female) with an opportunity to pursue a nursing education (Robinson, 1973). Despite these early efforts, men have remained underrepresented in nursing. A significant barrier to the recruitment of men into nursing has been a lack of awareness regarding the opportunities in nursing. Guidance counselors have little understanding of the range of positions that are available to nurses (Kelly et al., 1996; LaRocco, 2004). They routinely discourage intelligent students from nursing.

RECENT STUDIES

LaRocco's Study

LaRocco (2004) explored the process leading to a male nurse's decision to become a nurse and the advantages and disadvantages of nursing as a career for men, and attempted to identify policies and practices that facilitate both the entry of men into nursing and the retention of male nurses in the workforce. In a study using grounded theory methodology, 20 men nurses participated in semistructured, in-depth, individual interviews. The participants had 1–35 years of experience as RNs. Socializing men into nursing emerged from the data as the basic social process. This process includes a trajectory of four stages that encompasses the path men travel in becoming nurses. The stages occur in a linear manner. The first stage is *prior to considering nursing,* followed by *choosing nursing* and *becoming a nurse,* and ending with *being a nurse.* From this basic social process and from men's comments and suggestions about the recruitment and retention of men in nursing, LaRocco proposed recommendations for policies and practices that will facilitate the entry of men into nursing and will improve the retention of men in the workforce.

The first stage, *prior to considering nursing,* includes the time when the man was a high-school student. For 17 of the men, nursing was not seen as a career option during their adolescent years. The men emphatically reported that high-school counselors did not suggest nursing as a career. As for the two men who had gone to nursing school directly from high school, guidance counselors encouraged them to consider some other health profession, such as physical therapy.

The second stage of socializing men into nursing, *choosing nursing,* contains two themes: opportunities in nursing and family/social influences. By the time the men chose nursing, they had become aware of the variety of opportunities that existed within the profession. The opportunities mentioned by the men included job security, helping people, interacting with patients, and obtaining a potentially satisfying career. The second theme in the stage of choosing nursing was family/societal influences. Many of the men described close relatives who were nurses and considered them as positive influences on their choice of nursing as a career. The men also received encouragement from people in other health professions whom they worked with or knew. Most of the men received significant emotional support from family members. This was especially true for the men who graduated more recently (within the 10 years prior to the interviews). The men also reported that their friends reacted favorably to their career choice, although some were teased in a good-natured way.

The third stage in the process, *becoming a nurse,* encompasses the time when the men were in nursing school. Many of the participants did not think there were any hindrances to their successful completion of their basic nursing program. However, the behaviors of a few specific faculty members were described as negative factors during their educational program. In several instances these behaviors were not directed at the male student but were behaviors that would be perceived as negative by any student. Many of the men commented on a specific instructor whom they described as "excellent" or "phenomenal." While none of the men identified the lack of male nursing instructors as a hindrance, the four that did have male instructors were pleased to have people they considered as role models.

An important theme that emerged from the last stage, *being a nurse,* was that of nursing being a genderless profession. Although some of the men identified differences between men and women nurses, they did not see the profession of nursing as being more consistent with a female role. Half of the men strongly disliked the term male nurse. While most of the men did not view the term as derogatory, they thought it was antiquated or ridiculous. One participant did not think that the term was still in use, but this participant had spent his entire career in the military service, where men comprise approximately one-third of the nurses.

LaRocco (2004) also asked the men nurses to describe policies and practices that they thought would be influential in recruiting men into nursing and in retaining men currently working as nurses. The recruitment suggestions included educating the public about the positive aspects of nursing as a career and exposing children to men who are nurses. Many of the men thought that the general public lacks an understanding of the role of the nurse and the many opportunities available to nurses. The specific positive aspects of nursing about which the men thought the public should be educated included salaries, job security and flexibility, and the opportunities available for career progression and specialty practice. Many of the men also indicated the need for a visible presence of men in nursing. They felt that it is important for young men to meet men who are nurses and to hear men discuss nursing as rewarding. All of the men said they would encourage other men to consider nursing as a career.

Twelve of the men nurses indicated that many retention strategies were not specific to men. Their suggestions for the retention of all nurses of either gender included the provision of adequate salaries and benefits, a good practice environment, and personal recognition. Half of the men mentioned money as an important aspect in retaining nurses. One man favorably described the four-step clinical ladder that his employing institution had developed. In this program, expertise and knowledge are recognized. Each step on the ladder includes a 5% increase in base salary. He thought this opportunity for salary growth while remaining at the bedside would help to stem the migration of nurses into management. A good practice environment was described as a place where employees were treated with respect and dignity and given control over nursing practice. Personal recognition programs did not have to include the receipt of "a gold Rolex," but rather some smaller token such as less shift rotation.

The Bernard Hodes Study

The Bernard Hodes Group (2005) conducted a study in conjunction with the California Institute for Nursing and Healthcare and the Coalition for Nursing Careers in California, in which men nurses were asked to identify the best vehicles to attract men to nursing. Using a 0–5 scale in which a response of 5 indicated the highest level of importance, the participants responded that more knowledgeable career counselors was the most important (mean score of 4.42). Other responses in which the mean exceeded a score of 4 included school visits/male nurse presentations (4.40), shadow programs (4.10), ads in men's magazines (4.09), the use of ads similar to those in the recent campaign by Johnson & Johnson in which men nurses were prominently featured alongside female nurses (4.04), and the placement of ads in sports magazines (4.02). The men were also asked to identify key talking points for communicating themes of men in nursing to students. These included discussing nursing in an inclusive, non-gender-specific message; describing nursing as providing stable employment; discussing the multiple areas of clinical nursing practice; and describing nurses as highly skilled and having autonomy. The men also described the types of images that would best convey the message of men in nursing to males. These images included action/military, high-tech, and physical diversity scenes, and the depiction of nurses as heroes and team players. The men emphasized the use of real nurses as opposed to actors or models. The images that they did not want to see portrayed as representative of men in nursing included gender stereo-types (homosexuality, effeminacy, or machismo) and images of nurses as glorified maids or orderlies, nurses as subservient to physicians, or nurses in white uniforms in unidentified clinical settings.

The participants in the study were also asked to describe the meth-od of taking the message that men can be nurses to students in various age groups. While a few participants felt that elementary-school chil-dren were too young to appreciate the message that men can be nurses, many participants offered very concrete suggestions on how to address students in general. Some indicated that they had already participated in activities at local elementary schools, including classroom visits and career-day programs. The suggestions for taking the message of nursing as a career for men to middle/junior-school students included field trips and hands-on events (such as taking blood pressures, listening to heart sounds) as well as shadow programs. As far as high-school students were concerned, the respondents suggested that boys at this stage would be ready to receive more detailed information about nursing programs, ad-mission requirements, and scholarships. Overall, exposure to men who are nurses and having men nurses discuss what they do on the job, with an emphasis on technology and saving lives, were seen as ways to change the stereotypical view that only women could or should be nurses.

STRATEGIES FOR RECRUITING MEN INTO NURSING

Based on recent research and on the opinions of other men who are nurses ("Where Are the Men?" 2003), many strategies have been identified to increase the number of men in the workforce. Educational institutions, health care employers, professional nursing and health care organizations, and the government all have a role in working to ensure the continued supply of an adequate number of nurses to meet the increasing demands of our aging population. The strategies to be considered include the follow-ing: exposing young male students to men nurses who have had successful and satisfying careers in nursing so that they can see nursing as a possible career; educating high-school guidance counselors about nursing so they can speak knowledgeably about it as a career option for adoles-cent boys and girls; improving the public's image of nursing to more accurately reflect what nurses really do; focusing on the flexibility and job security that nursing provides; de-emphasizing the female nurturing values and highlighting the professional aspects of nursing; producing nursing-school brochures and Web sites that show men in active nurs-ing roles; advertising nursing programs in places where young boys and men will see them; providing competitive salaries for nurses; providing flexible and accelerated nursing-education programs that appeal to the man pursuing a second career; and creating a male-friendly environment for men who have entered nursing school, by providing mentoring of male students by male faculty or by encouraging the men to meet informally or formally by forming a chapter of the American Assembly for Men in Nursing (a professional nursing organization that has the recruitment of men into nursing as one of its stated goals).

Many of the points described above have been considered and incorporated into creative media programs designed to recruit men into nursing. Examples of these programs include the Oregon Center for Nursing's "Man Enough to Be a Nurse" campaign and calendars featuring men nurses from the Nebraska Hospital Association and the Mississippi Hospital Association's Health Career Center. These specific programs are discussed in detail in chapter 14. However, research is needed to explore the effectiveness of these and various other media-based recruitment programs.

Many health care institutions and nursing schools have encouraged male nurses to attend career days or gender diversity programs at local schools. These programs provide an opportunity for boys to talk to a male nurse and hear at first hand about nursing and the work that nurses do. Pictures of men nurses in action help to dispel the myth that nursing is focused on assisting clients with personal hygiene tasks. A formal program to expose young boys to men who are nurses has been presented on the campus of the University of South Carolina in Columbia. Thirty-seven seventh- and eighth-grade boys attended a five-day program called MENS CAMP (Males Exploring Nursing in South Carolina—Altering Middle School Perceptions). The boys were taught technical skills including setting up IVs and suturing. A college representative also met with the boys to discuss academic requirements and to provide information about the admission exams that would be required to enter the university. Follow-up calls to the students, and later to their parents, to educate them about nursing as a career were included in the program. Each boy received a T-shirt with the program logo and a slogan reading "I could be a nurse by 2010."

Dispelling stereotypes about nursing is one way to make nursing seem more male friendly. To accomplish this, the University of Nebraska Medical Center College of Nursing made changes in its informational brochures and marketing approaches (D. Williams, 2002). The redesign replaced the pink and teal colors previously used in the brochures with reds and blacks. Using bolder, simpler type styles instead of a fancy script also provided a more masculine look. The photographs included in the marketing materials were more gender diverse, with men shown in fast-paced clinical settings.

Some schools of nursing have a significantly higher percentage of men students than others, rising as high as 40% at Excelsior College in New York State (American Association of Colleges of Nursing, 2005a). Excelsior College describes itself as an educational institution designed to deliver college education to adults online at a pace congruent with their busy schedules (Excelsior College, 2005). The flexibility and self-pacing of the program allows students to meet family and work commitments while pursuing their nursing education. This model tends to be more attractive to adult learners and may be particularly attractive to men, who often enter nursing at an older age than do women (Galbraith, 1991; Marsland, Robinson, and Murrells, 1996; Okrainec, 1994; Winson, 1992). However, other schools attract a relatively high percentage of male nursing students to their generic (entry-level) baccalaureate programs without making any special recruitment efforts directed at men. These include the University of South Alabama (18.9%; Davis, personal communication, 2005), the University of Texas at Tyler (18.4%; Pam Martin, personal communication, 2005), and Nicholls State University (15.4%; Sue Westerbrook, personal communication, 2005). While the schools may not be employing any planned effort to specifically recruit men into their programs, there may be local community influences that are working to increase the percentage of men in their programs. Research examining why these schools are attracting higher numbers of male students is warranted.

Scholarships for male nursing students are another means of providing support to men who are pursuing a career in nursing. In 2005, with money provided by the Johnson & Johnson Foundation, the foundation arm of the American Assembly for Men in Nursing provided seven scholarships for pre-licensure men and three for men who were pursuing graduate nursing studies. These scholarships were unique among all the scholarships available to nursing students in that they specifically targeted men.

CONCLUSION

Improved recruitment and retention of men in nursing will strengthen the profession and help to provide the diversity necessary to enhance patient care, while providing men with the opportunity of career satisfaction. At a time of an impending nursing shortage, any actions that exclude half of the potential candidates for nursing careers will be detrimental to the future health of our society. The utilization of multiple strategies to encourage men and boys to view nursing as a career option and to provide support for male nursing students as they pursue their education should be urgently addressed by the nursing profession. Until men represent half of our entering nursing classes, all nurses and health care policymakers should continue to focus on strategies designed to aggressively recruit and retain men in nursing.

REFERENCES

American Association of Colleges of Nursing. (2005a). *Nursing faculty shortage fact sheet.* Retrieved October 9, 2005, from http://www.aacn.nche.edu/Media/pdf/FacultyShortageFactSheet.pdf.

American Association of Colleges of Nursing. (2005b, Fall). *Schools of nursing with the highest proportion of male students, generic (entry-level) baccalaureate programs: Special report to the American Assembly for Men in Nursing.* Washington, DC: Author.

Barkley, T. W., & Kohler, E. A. (1992). Is nursing's image a deterrent to recruiting men into the profession? Male high school students respond. *Nursing Forum, 27*(2), 9–14.

Bernard Hodes Group. (2005). *Men in nursing study.* Retrieved October 3, 2005, from http://www.hodes.com/healthcarematters/pdfs/meninnursing2005.pdf

Boughn, S. (1994). Why do men choose nursing? *Nursing and Health Care, 15,* 406–411.

Buerhaus, P. I., Staiger, D. O., & Auerbach, D. I. (2004, November 17). New signs of a strengthening U.S. nurse labor market? *Health Affairs (Web Exclusive).* Retrieved April 5, 2005, from http://content.healthaffairs.org/cgi/content/full/hthaff.w4.526/DCI

Bullough, V. L. (1994). Men, women, and nursing history. *Journal of Professional Nursing 10*(3), 127.

Bullough, V. L. (1997). Men in nursing: Problems and prospects. In J. C. McCloskey & H. K. Grace (Eds.), *Current issues in nursing* (5th ed., pp. 589–594). St. Louis, MO: Mosby.

Bullough, V. L. (2001). Finally we have arrived: Men in nursing. In J. M. Dochterman & H. K. Grace (Eds.), *Current issues in nursing* (6th ed., pp. 504–511). St. Louis, MO: Mosby.

Bush, P. J. (1976). The male nurse: A challenge to traditional role identities. *Nursing Forum, 15,* 390–405.

Canadian Nurses Association. (2003). *Registered nurses 2003: Statistical highlights.* Retrieved April 23, 2005, from http://canaiic.ca/CAN/nursing/statistics/2002highlights/default_e.aspx

Christman, L. (1974). Let's have more men in nursing. *Nursing, 4*(5), 16–17.

Evans, J. (1997). Men in nursing: Issues of gender segregation and hidden advantage. *Journal of Advanced Nursing, 26*(2), 226–231.

Evans, J. (2004) Men nurses: A historical and feminist perspective. *Journal of Advanced Nursing, 47,* 321–328.

Excelsior College. (2005). *About Excelsior College.* Retrieved October 2, 2005, from https://www.excelsior.edu/portal/page?_pageid=57,35974&_dad=portal&_schema=PORTAL

Galbraith, M. (1991). Attracting men to nursing: What will they find important in their career? *Journal of Nursing Education, 30,* 182–186.

German Nurses Association. (2004). *A few facts about the German Nurses Association.* Retrieved April 25, 2005, from http://www.dbfk.de/englishnew.htm

Gorman, D. (2003). A nurse by any other name ... *Nursing Spectrum, 7*(10), 10. [northeast edition.]

Gray, D. P., Kramer, M., Minick, P., McGehee, L., Thomas, D., & Greiner, D. (1996). Heterosexism in nursing education. *Journal of Nursing Education, 35,* 204–210.

Halloran, E. J., & Welton, J. M. (1994). Why aren't there more men in nursing? In J. C. McCloskey & H. K. Grace (Eds.), *Current Issues in Nursing* (4th ed., 683–691). St. Louis, MO: Mosby.

Health Resources and Services Administration. (2004). The registered nurse population: National sample survey of registered nurses—Preliminary findings. Retrieved February 28, 2006 from ftp://ftp.hrsa.gov/bhpr/nursing/rnpopulation/the_registered_nurse_population.pdf

International Council of Nurses. (2004). *Nursing workforce profile.* Retrieved April 20, 2005, from http://www.icn.ch/SewDatasheet04.pdf

Kelly, N. R., Shoemaker, M., & Steele, T. (1996). The experience of being a male student nurse. *Journal of Nursing Education, 35,* 170–174.

LaRocco, S. A. (2004). *Policies and practices that influence recruitment and retention of men in nursing: A grounded theory study of socializing men into nursing.* Unpublished doctoral dissertation, University of Massachusetts, Boston.

London, F. (1987). Should men be actively recruited into nursing? *Nursing Administration Quarterly, 12,* 75–81.

Mackintosh, C. (1997). A historical study of men in nursing. *Journal of Advanced Nursing, 26,* 232–236.

MacPhail, J. (1996). Men in nursing. In J. R. Kerr & J. MacPhail (Eds.), *Canadian nursing: Issues and perspectives* (3rd ed., pp. 74–81). St. Louis MO: Mosby.

Mangan, E. (1994). Private lives. *Nursing Times, 90*(14), 60–64.

Marsland, L., Robinson, S., & Murrells, T. (1996). Pursuing a career in nursing: Differences between men and women qualifying as registered general nurses. *Journal of Nursing Management, 4,* 231–241.

Nightingale, F. (1860). *Notes on nursing: What it is and what it is not.* New York: Dover.

Okrainec, G. D. (1994). Perceptions of nursing education held by male nursing students. *Western Journal of Nursing Research, 16,* 94–107.

Poliafico, J. K. (1998). Nursing's gender gap. *RN, 61*(10), 39–42.

Rallis, S. (1990). I want to be a nurse, not a stereotype. *RN, 53*(4), 160.

Robinson, A. M. (1973). Men in nursing: Their career goals and image are changing. *RN,* 36–41.

Ryan, S., & Porter, S. (1993). Men in nursing: A cautionary comparative critique. *Nursing Outlook, 41,* 262–267.

Spratley, E., Johnson, A., Sochalski, J., Fritz, M., & Spencer, W. (2001). *The registered nurse population March 2000: Findings from the National Sample Survey of Registered Nurses.* Washington, DC: U.S. Department of Health and Human Services, Health Resources and Services Administration.

Sullivan, E. J. (2000). Men in nursing: The importance of gender diversity. *Journal of Professional Nursing, 16,* 253–254.

Villeneuve, M. J. (1994). Recruiting and retaining men in nursing: A review of the literature. *Journal of Professional Nursing, 10,* 217–228.

Where are the men? (2003). *Nursing, 33*(7), 43–45.

Williams, C. L. (1992). The glass escalator: Hidden advantages for men in the "female" professions. *Social Problems, 39*(3), 253–268.

Williams, C. L. (1995). Hidden advantages for men in nursing. *Nursing Administration Quarterly, 19,* 63–70.

Williams, D. (2002, Spring). Looking for a few good men. *Minority Nurse,* 22–27.

Winson, G. (1992). A study of nurse career paths. *Senior Nurse, 12*(3), 11–14, 19.

CHAPTER FOURTEEN

Are You Man Enough to Be a Nurse? Challenging Male Nurse Media Portrayals and Stereotypes

Deborah A. Burton and Terry R. Misener

INTRODUCTION

In order to address the growing nursing shortage in Oregon, the Oregon Center for Nursing (OCN) in 2002 mounted an aggressive campaign aimed at informing the public of the need for nurses and the advantages for those interested in health careers to explore nursing. Given that gender is one of the most significant demographic imbalances in nursing, it became evident that recruiting from the virtually untapped male population needed to be an essential component of a campaign to reverse the shortage. Considering that nurses are continually displeased with media images of the nursing profession, especially images of men in nursing, the OCN designed a targeted, positive media and recruitment campaign. Relevant media and literature were examined, as were prevailing stereotypes of both nurses in general, and men who were nurses were specifically analyzed. The campaign was then launched with two primary objectives: recruit men into nursing and correct inaccurate public images of men in nursing. This chapter will discuss how negative media images of men in nursing have hampered the recruitment of men into nursing and how the current campaign and similar strategies can improve recruitment by providing alternative images of men in nursing.

255

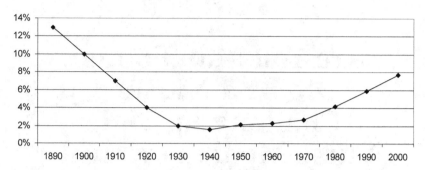

FIGURE 14.1   Percentage of self-identified male nurses in the U.S. nursing workforce, 1890–2000. Source: U.S. Census Bureau and U.S. Bureau of Labor Statistics, provided by Washington University, 2004.

BACKGROUND

The number of men who identified themselves as nurses in U.S. Census Bureau figures fluctuated between a high of approximately 13% in 1890 and a low of less than 2% in 1940. Slowly the percentage has increased to almost 8% in 2000 (Washington University, 2004). This trend is summarized graphically in Figure 14.1. While the overall proportion of men in the profession does not approach the percentage of men in the general population, the growth from 2.7% in 1970 to almost 8% in 2000 represents a 300% increase.

In response to the mid-1980s shortage, Department of Health and Human Services (DHHS) Secretary Otis Bowen, MD, in 1987, commissioned a comprehensive study on the state of the nursing profession. The Secretary's Commission on Nursing (DHHS, 1988) provided 16 major recommendations, one of which appealed to the profession to "establish a national campaign to promote the image of men in nursing and the idea of nursing as an attractive career option for men…[and]…to ensure the accurate portrayal of nursing in entertainment and news programs" (DHHS, 1998, p. 44). The profession failed to undertake this campaign, presumably because it was not a priority for the 96%-female nurse workforce at the time. For another 20 years, essentially nothing happened to increase the recruitment of men into the profession or to address inaccurate public images and stereotypes of male nurses. This failure has persisted, despite numerous articles and debates on the issue and multiple resolutions by major nursing organizations calling for solutions to the problem of the underparticipation of men in nursing.

Beyond the fact that the vast majority of nurse leaders and decision makers have been women, additional factors can help explain why men have remained such a small minority in nursing. Some attribute the collective lack of recruitment efforts to the perceived advantages enjoyed by male nurses as a token minority group, accorded special privileges that reflect their inherent gender-based desire for power (Kleinman, 2004; Neighbours, 2005). Others cite discrimination within the profession itself as having prevented the emergence of a uniform strategy to reverse trends in male underrepresentation in nursing. From these perspectives, nursing has not been willing to correct the gender imbalance, as it would erode women's power base in the profession. Any masculine characteristics inherent in nursing have been devalued, and as a result, the profession has suffered (Burtt, 1998; Porter-O'Grady, 2003b). Irrespective of why these problems have persisted, the present nursing-shortage crisis requires the aggressive embracing and encouraging of *any* potential source of qualified new nurse recruits, especially men and minorities.

MALE NURSE STEREOTYPES AND PUBLIC IMAGES

Stereotypes are generalizations or assumptions made about a group's members, based on an image of what people in the group are like (Burgess, 2003). Media portrayals can powerfully perpetuate stereotypes. In contrast with the wide, though inaccurate, range of media portrayals of female nurses, male nurses are rarely depicted (AAN, 1983; Cunningham, 1999). However, male nurse depictions have perpetuated negative stereotypes that can be categorized into four themes. The first is the "physician wanna-be" or "failed medical school applicant." This stereotype stems from inaccurate historical depictions of nursing as passive, unintelligent work. The presumption is that any man would prefer to be a physician and that nursing is an unfortunate career choice, resulting from lack of intelligence and/or nonmasculine attributes. In the film *Meet the Parents* (Vincent & Roach, 2001), Ben Stiller plays the part of a nurse whose interactions with his fiancée's family illustrate these themes.

The second category is "gay/effeminate." As in any profession, gay men work as nurses. However, there is no evidence that the number of gay men in nursing is disproportionate to the population in general. In *Meet the Parents* (Vincent & Roach, 2001), Ben Stiller's character must face his father-in-law's criticism that nursing is effeminate. The general stereotype is that men who choose nursing must be both gay and effeminate since they have chosen a career in so-called women's work.

The third category is "misfit." This stereotype is portrayed in the 1945 classic, *The Lost Weekend* (Brackett, Jackson, & Wilder, 1945). In this film, an alcoholic is forced into a detoxification ward and is attended by a ghoulish, spooky, effeminate male nurse character played by Frank Faylen. Another example is the odd male nurse character, played by Phillip Seymour Hoffman, who attends a dying man in the 1999 film *Magnolia* (Anderson et al., 2000). These nurses are presumed to be hiding in nursing because they are odd and do not fit into mainstream male occupations.

The fourth category is "womanizer." This stereotype was illustrated in one episode of the emergency department television sitcom *Scrubs* (Allen et al., 2001). In this episode, Rick Schroeder made a guest appearance as a very masculine nurse who caught the eye of a female physician (although later episodes cast him in a more positive and accurate light). The presumption is that heterosexual men choose nursing for sexual exploits and conquest or as a means to advance professionally on the backs of less ambitious female nurses (Berry, 2004; Center for Nursing Advocacy, 2003a, 2003b; Icon, 2004; Rasmussen, 2001).

Effects on the Nursing Profession

Evidence abounds that the negative and inaccurate public images of nurses have had long-term, deleterious effects on the profession (Berry, 2004; Burtt, 1998; Center for Nursing Advocacy, 2003b; DHHS, 1988; Kleinman, 2004; McRae, 2003; Porter-O'Grady 2003b; Sochalski, 2002; C. Williams, 1983). Not only do media images reinforce inaccurate, outdated, and unprofessional images of nurses in the public eye, but these images directly influence both a nurse's self-perception and the profession's ability to advance and evolve. For men, this is doubly problematic since not only are male nurse stereotypes inaccurate but male nurses are often lost in the overwhelmingly female archetypes and characterizations of the nurse as female (D. Williams, 2003). According to Porter-O'Grady (2003b),

> All kinds of images emerge when conflicting mental pictures roll out and create perceptual and experiential dissonance between what "should be" and what is. Interestingly enough, when the man is the nurse, many frames of reference emerge that would not be applied in reference to a woman who is a nurse. Comments related to competence ("What's wrong, couldn't you get into medical school?"); intelligence (You're a bright guy, why'd you become a nurse?"); sexual identity (Are you gay or something?"); and a host of others indicate the prevalent disparity in perception between being a man and a nurse. All indicate that there must be something not quite right with a man's choice of nursing as a career. (p. 1)

If the nursing profession is to embrace diversity in its ranks, such that the composition of the profession mirrors the composition of the patient population, these pervasive, inaccurate stereotypes must be addressed and changed.

Reversing Negative Stereotypes

In general, correcting long-term stereotypes takes both individual and collective action. Over the past 20 years, the nursing profession has made significant progress in aggressively attacking negative media images. Nurses Media Watch, the Center for Nursing Advocacy, and the British Nursing the Future organize public media campaigns aimed at analyzing media depictions of nurses. These organizations direct massive political and public pressure toward television and film producers in cases where portrayals of nurses are deemed negative and inaccurate (Berry 2004; Center for Nursing Advocacy, 2004).

As the worst nursing shortage yet gathered steam in 2000, J. W. Thompson (JWT) Communications conducted focus groups involving over 1,800 high-school students across the United States (LeMaire, 2004; Sherman, 2000). The JWT focus groups were aimed at shaping marketing campaigns to recruit bright, promising young people away from other career choices and into nursing.

In this project, JWT asked the students about their impressions of nursing as a career choice. In general, high-school students reported getting many of their impressions of nursing from television shows, such as *E.R.* (Chulack, Woodward et al., 1994). Boys described nursing as "girls' work," a lowly career choice, and very task oriented, "like shop classes." Information gleaned from these focus groups led to the largest public media nursing recruitment campaign ever, the Johnson & Johnson "Dare to Care" ad campaign.

Johnson & Johnson in 2001 underwrote and launched a $30-million sustained media and public awareness campaign aimed at marketing nursing as a challenging and rewarding career. Many of the actors in its television ads were men from a range of ethnic backgrounds. The ads have been consistently shown at prime time, for example, during the 2002 Winter and 2004 Summer Olympics. Nursing is represented as challenging, rewarding, intellectually stimulating and well compensated. Other features of the campaign include the development of focused nursing career Web sites, recruitment materials, and videos, large public events, and media packets (Johnson & Johnson, 2002).

THE OREGON EXPERIENCE

In 2002, the Oregon Center for Nursing (OCN), a state-based nurse workforce center, was charged with increasing the proportion of men and ethnic minorities in the Oregon nurse workforce. Although men comprise almost 12% of the Oregon RN workforce, 50% representation is the long-term goal of the Oregon State Board of Nursing (OSBN, personal communication, 2004). In partnership with a major university in Oregon, focus groups of middle- and high-school boys were convened; these groups revealed that Johnson & Johnson's efforts were having little to no effect on "stereotypic" boys interested in health careers. Stereotypic high-school boys can be defined as those who embody prevailing male stereotypes: for example, risk takers, adventurers, competitors, logical thinkers, leaders, protectors, and aggressors (Femiano & Nickerson, 1989). When asked why the Johnson & Johnson ads were not having the desired effect, the resounding response from such boys was, "Oh, [male nurses], they're all gay" (University of Portland, 2003).

Other focus groups, of middle- and high-school guidance counselors from across the state, were also convened (University of Portland, 2003). When asked how better to connect with typical male and ethnic minority students, the counselors agreed the answer was to find nurses that "looked like the target audience—nurses with whom the students could directly connect and relate." Other focus groups conducted with male nursing students revealed a need to emphasize the more masculine aspects of nursing, and to drop the term male nurse. Many student participants cited having a nurse as close family member or friend as pivotal in their career choice. Others had positive nurse role models who were men or who came from the military where nurses are highly respected as officers. A number chose nursing for the salary and job security.

In Oregon, it was clear that reversing nursing's negative public image was going to take collective public action, combined with one-on-one interaction with each potential male recruit. The target audience for the OCN project was stereotypic Oregon male high-school students with academic potential and interest in a health-related career. Although many men enter nursing as a second career, young men were targeted due to their potential for a long-term career commitment to nursing. Nursing's image needed to be repackaged and marketed for this young male audience. With the help of a seasoned communications consultant, it became clear that Oregon needed to discard the usual strategies for recruiting men into nursing. The materials being used at the time were either gender neutral or heavily feminine, especially in the use of female images and pastel colors. Porter-O'Grady (2003a) validated the OCN marketing strategy in remarks made in an interview on whether nursing could ever overcome its male-nurse-related issues, by stating that

> A national campaign to recruit men should feature images of men
> performing action-oriented, fast-paced nursing tasks. Anything that

moves away from a passive image of men in nursing and the work they do will grab the attention of contemporary men. We should also raise the visibility of articulate professional men holding powerful leadership positions in professional organizations. (p. 2)

OCN simply needed to adopt proven and effective targeted marketing principles. The communications consultant helped refine the messages to the young men, for example, "nursing takes courage and technical skill"; "nursing is challenging, fast-paced and never dull"; and "nursing offers unlimited opportunity, good pay and job security for life." However, in order for young men to hear these messages, OCN first had to grab their attention.

The Oregon In-Your-Face Strategy: "Are You Man Enough to Be a Nurse?"

Armed with the marketing messages, boys, counselors, and male nursing students had given us, and our awareness of what was *not* working, OCN set out to change the public image of men as nurses. First, practicing male nurses were recruited who (a) embodied stereotypic male characteristics (athletic prowess, masculine avocations, and military accomplishments); (b) looked stereotypically male; (c) chose nursing and loved their nursing role; (d) represented a wide range of ethnicities, ages, and nursing practice roles; and (e) could articulate the fact that being male was very compatible with their nursing role and that they were very satisfied with their chosen career.

Next, a theme that would captivate attention had to be selected. "Are You Man Enough to Be a Nurse?" seemed the perfect theme. The communications consultant and a photographer worked to project the desired visual image of men as nurses: strong, powerful, caring, self-assured, confident, smart, successful, technically astute, and very masculine. The photographer insisted that in order to advance a powerful, masculine message, we needed to use black and white photography and we should not allow the men to smile. A large, bold, black font was selected for extra impact (see Figure 14.2).

The campaign passed a marketing litmus test when a draft was presented to members of the targeted adolescent male audience. When asked for their reactions, their consistent response was, "*No way* are those guys nurses!" The poster had hit the mark. At one university where the poster was placed on a bulletin board outside a professor's office, the professor was continually struck by the number of men who walked by the poster, stopped, backed up, and concentrated more fully on the image. Obviously, it got attention.

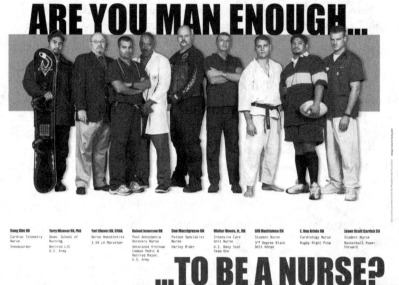

FIGURE 14.2   "Are You Man Enough to Be a Nurse?" poster. Male
nursing recruitment poster featuring nine practicing Oregon nurses
with a variety of masculine-related accomplishments in sports and in
the military. © Oregon Center for Nursing, by permission.

Overcoming Persistent, Inaccurate Stereotypes in Oregon

The permanent replacement of long-term, negative stereotypes does not
happen with one application or one campaign. In Oregon, saturation
techniques have been used to reach the public repetitively to reinforce a
new image. First, the poster was mailed to every middle-school and high-
school guidance counselor in Oregon, with a letter highlighting the reasons why talented young people with an interest in health careers should
be directed to nursing. The packet included nursing recruitment and educational resource materials.

Next, a very aggressive media campaign instantly launched the male-
nurse theme into the public eye. The men depicted in the poster made
visits to high-school and community groups. To give interested high-
school boys an opportunity to experience nursing at first hand, a daylong
Saturday course, "Men in Scrubs," was created. The course is offered
through a local nonprofit occupational-immersion program, known
as the "Saturday Academy." "Men in Scrubs" is taught exclusively by

practicing men nurses, and it includes clinical and simulated laboratory time and shadow experiences with practicing male nurses.

Sponsorship from Providence Health System, Oregon's largest health care system, supported the placement of the digital image of the poster everywhere imaginable. Soon the "Are You Man Enough?" poster image was on the backs of transit buses, on billboards in rural areas, and on the sides of urban commuter trains. The Portland VA Medical Center reproduced the image on a recruitment postcard. Other facilities used it on placemats in hospital cafeterias. The poster was sent to every legislator involved in health-related legislation, and to the library of every college that had a nursing program.

Soon thereafter, Silverton Hospital, located in rural Oregon, adopted the "male reality" theme by developing its own local version of the poster (Figure 14.3). The Silverton image highlighted men from all departments in the hospital who were nurses. This revised poster was used to promote the hospital as an employer of choice, and to support nursing recruitment in the local community. Later, in 2003, Providence Health System supported the creation of a digital video spot that animated the poster, setting it to music with voice-over messages. This clip was played at Portland-area movie theatres that featured films marketed to adolescents.

Next, OCN aligned with the Virginia Partnership for Nursing (VPN), the State of Virginia's nursing workforce and promotion center. Virginia was experiencing similar male image and recruitment challenges. OCN negotiated the rights for Virginia to use the Oregon men and the

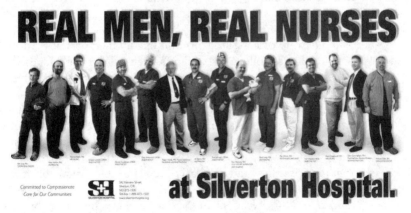

FIGURE 14.3   Silverton Hospital (Oregon) recruitment poster featuring male nurses employed by the hospital. © Silverton Hospital, by permission.

"Are You Man Enough to Be a Nurse?" slogan. Soon the Virginia version of the slogan, "Man Enough to Be a Nurse," appeared on the East coast in athletic arenas and sports programs, and in middle and high schools. OCN then partnered with VPN on another project, targeting younger children. With support from the Bernard Hodes Group, *Nurses with Rocket Shoes,* a coloring book that featured men nurses as superheroes, was jointly produced and released.

MEN NURSES IN *SPORTS ILLUSTRATED:* IS IT POSSIBLE?

Throughout this campaign, OCN consistently kept the men in nursing theme alive in the Oregon media. Soon the poster had also appeared in 28 non-Oregon nursing and health care publications in four countries. However, *all* expectations were exceeded when, with help from Bernard Hodes and the Virginia Partnership for Nursing, the Oregon men appeared in a full-page ad in the East coast version of *Sports Illustrated* (2003), seen in Figure 14.4.

INNOVATIONS IN OTHER STATES

As Oregon saturation strategies have taken hold, other states and programs have launched initiatives to repackage men's image in nursing. *None* of these efforts remotely resemble traditional nurse recruitment efforts. Some innovative examples include the following:

- *Iowa:* A group of male students and faculty members at the University of Iowa College of Nursing's Men in Nursing Mentoring Task Force developed an entire project, Web site, and recruitment materials focusing on a positive experience for men in nursing school. It features real experiences of male nursing students and faculty. While there was no communication between Oregon and the leaders of the Iowa project during its design, it is interesting to note how closely the two graphic representations mirror each other in appearance and emphasis (see Figure 14.5, available from http://www.nursing.uiowa.edu/students/men.pdf).
- *Nebraska:* Nurse leaders in Nebraska were intrigued by the Oregon project but concluded that stereotypic men in Nebraska looked very little like Oregon men, either in ethnicity or in avocation. The Nebraska Hospital Association collaborated to release a spectacular all-male nursing calendar in 2004, with

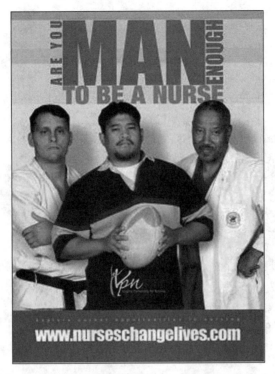

FIGURE 14.4   *Sports Illustrated* full-page advertisement developed by Bernard Hodes, Virginia Partnership for Nursing, and Oregon Center for Nursing. © Bernard Hodes, Oregon Center for Nursing, by permission.

each month featuring a practicing male nurse. The stereotypic Nebraska men include football players, weight lifters, farmers, and bow hunters. Subsequently, challenged by a looming severe shortage at a time when only 4.2% of the state's nurses were male, the hospital association developed a male-only nursing scholarship program (see http://www.nhanet.org/publications/workforce).

- *Mississippi:* Nearly simultaneous with the Nebraska project, the Mississippi Hospital Association produced an all-male nursing calendar featuring the real-life stories of Mississippi's practicing men nurses. An accompanying campaign focused on recruitment and career information (see http://www.mshealthcareers.com/calendar).
- *Texas:* A group of men nursing students at the University of Texas have formed the Longhorn Association of Men in Nursing.

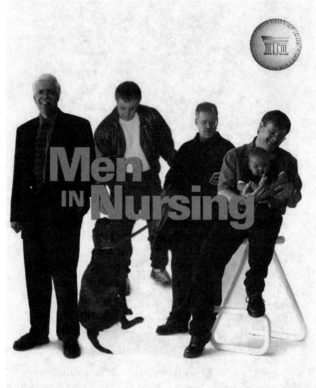

FIGURE 14.5   University of Iowa College of Nursing poster.
© University of Iowa College of Nursing, by permission.

Its mission is to foster nursing education, facilitate unity among
future colleagues and leaders in nursing, encourage men to
consider nursing as a career, and promote a positive image of
men in the field of nursing (see http://www.nur.utexas.edu/
MeninNsg/index.html).

- *Washington:* The University of Washington School of Nursing
  has a dedicated Web page of resources for men in nursing. The
  Web page features the Oregon poster, along with a companion
  poster, titled "Caring Knows No Boundaries," aimed at recruiting
  minorities into nursing (see http://www.son.washington.edu/
  students/min/).
- *Miscellaneous:* A nurse entrepreneur, Kathy Quan, has been marketing Father's Day gifts nationally for fathers who are nurses.

Promoted as "Is Your Dad a Nurse?" these gifts are available year-round (see http://nursing.about.com/od/nursesaroundtheworld/a/giftsformalenur.htm). Also, in 2002, the online magazine, *Male Nurse*, was launched to focus on issues facing men in nursing and to target recruitment and education (see http://www.malenursemagazine.com/about.htm).

EVALUATION

It is too soon to detect true increases in the number of men in the Oregon nursing ranks as a direct result of the saturation campaign, since the targeted audience is currently in school. However, if the 10-fold increase in the volume of e-mails and phone calls from interested men and parents of high-school boys following the release of the poster is any indication, a 40-to-80 year-old image glacier is beginning to thaw in Oregon and around the country. More tangible however, is the national online survey of male nurses conducted in 2004 by the Bernard Hodes Group, in conjunction with the California Institute for Nursing and the American Assembly for Men in Nursing (Bernard Hodes Group, 2005). The purpose was to more clearly identify the reasons underlying the small percentage of men in nursing. A total of 468 men participated in the survey (93% RNs, 7% nursing students; the average age was 44). A segment of the survey was dedicated to evaluating the impact of the Oregon poster, and to comparing its effectiveness with the Virginia Partnership for Nursing Project, "Man Enough to Be a Nurse" (which also appeared in *Sports Illustrated*; see Figure 14.4).

In the survey, respondents strongly preferred the Oregon poster over the Bernard Hodes/Virginia campaign. Specifically, on a 0 to 5 scale, the Oregon poster was rated higher in representing nursing as a challenging and responsible profession (3.52 vs. 2.63), representing nursing as a realistic career choice for men (3.62 vs. 2.84), and depicting a profession where men can learn and grow (3.44 vs. 2.53). Fully 91% rated the Oregon poster as most appealing overall to a male audience. The Oregon poster was rated highest in all creative element categories evaluated: Attention Getting, Informative, Believable, and Relevant.

According to the study authors, "There was an almost visceral reaction" to the two ads evaluated (Bernard Hodes, 2005, p. 39). There were numerous strongly negative narrative comments about both ads. Many respondents commented that the macho image was overemphasized, thus paradoxically reinforcing the stereotype that men in nursing are overwhelmingly gay or that nursing is not a masculine career option. One participant compared the message in both ads to asking, "Are you woman enough to be a doctor?" (p. 39). Each of these themes has also emerged in Oregon as the poster has become well known. Respondents in the Bernard Hodes survey identified the following types of images that would best convey men in nursing messages to males: "Action/military images," "Diversity," "Nurse as hero," "No actors," "Teamwork," and "High-tech." Key talking points for working with students were reported to be "Non-gender-specific messages," "Stable employment," "Multiple areas of practice," "Highly skilled," and "Autonomy" (Bernard Hodes, 2005).

IMAGINING LONG-TERM SUCCESS

Taken together, multiple innovations, focused initiatives, and the committed efforts of men who are nurses should result in a major improvement in gender balance in the nursing profession. In Oregon, success will be measured partially by a steady growth in new RN licenses issued to men. Specifically, OCN has evidence that saturation works and that the campaign is talking hold. Perhaps the greatest lesson is a simple Ringling Brothers/Barnum and Bailey Circus reminder: "If you want to train elephants, first you have to get their attention." Although aspects of the message have offended both men and women in nursing, the campaign got the public's attention, especially the attention of some formerly skeptical boys and their parents. The ongoing work of increasing the number of men in nursing has only just begun.

REFERENCES

Allen, G. (Producer/Director/Writer), et al. (2001). *Scrubs* [Television series]. New York: National Broadcasting Company.

Anderson, P. T. (Producer/Director/Writer), et al. (2000). *Magnolia* [Motion picture]. United States: New Line Cinema.

Bernard Hodes Group. (2005). *Men in nursing study.* Retrieved October 2, 2005, from http://www.hodes.com/healthcarematters/index.html

Berry, L. (2004). Is image important? *Nursing Standard, 18*(23), 14–16.

Brackett, C. (Producer/Writer), Jackson, C. R. (Writer), & Wilder, B. (Director/Writer). (1945). *The lost weekend* [Motion picture]. United States: Paramount Pictures.

Burgess, H. (2003). Stereotypes and characterization frames. *University of Colorado Conflict Resolution Consortium.* Retrieved October 2, 2005, from http://www.beyondintractability.org/m/stereotypes.jsp

Burtt, K. (1998). Male nurses still face bias. *American Journal of Nursing, 98*(9), 64-65.

Center for Nursing Advocacy. (2003a). *Men at work: Is "Scrubs" hurting or helping male nurses?* Retrieved October 2, 2005, from http://www.nursingadvocacy.org/news/2003jan30_scrubs.html

Center for Nursing Advocacy. (2003b). *NY Times: Men seen as one answer to nursing shortage.* Retrieved October 2, 2005, from http://www.nursingadvocacy.org/news/2003apr13_nyt.html

Center for Nursing Advocacy. (2004). *Why won't Hollywood fix its portrayal of nursing?* Retrieved October 2, 2005, from http://www.nursingadvocacy.org/faq/hollywood_behavior.html

Chulack, C., Woodward, L. (Executive Producers), et al. (1994). *E.R.* [Television series]. New York: National Broadcasting Company.

Cunningham, A. (1999). Nursing stereotypes. *Nursing Standard, 13*(45), 46–47.

Department of Health and Human Services (DHHS), Office of the Secretary. (1988). *Secretary's Commission on Nursing, Final Report.* Washington, DC: DHHS.

Femiano, S., & Nickerson, M. (1989, Fall). How do media images of men affect our lives? *Media & Values,* Issue No. 49.

Icon, E. (2004). Men in nursing today. *Working Nurse.* Retrieved October 2, 2005, from http://www.workingworld.com/magazine/viewarticle.asp?articleno=269&wn=1

Johnson & Johnson. (2002). *Campaign for nursing's future.* Retrieved October 2, 2005, from http://www.jnj.com/our_company/advertising/discover_nursing/index.htm

Kleinman, C. (2004). Understanding and capitalizing on men's advantages in nursing. *Journal of Nursing Administration, 34*(2), 78–82.

LeMaire, B. (2004). Sandy Summers, on media portrayal of nurses. *Nurseweek.* Retrieved October 2, 2005, from http://www.nurseweek.com/5min/SandySummers.asp

McRae, M. (2003). Men in obstetrical nursing: Perceptions of the role. *American Journal of Maternal-Child Nursing, 28*(3), 167–173.

Neighbours, C. (2005). Male nurses, men in a female dominated profession: The perceived need for masculinity maintenance. *AllNurses.Com.* Retrieved October 2, 2005 from http://www.allnurses.com/forums/showthread.php?t = 96304.

Porter-O'Grady, T. (2003a). Changing the imagery. *Nursing 2003, 33*(7), 43–44.

Porter-O'Grady, T. (2003b). *Nursing and the challenge of gender inequality.* Retrieved October 2, 2005, from http://www.nursingsociety.org/about/diversity_art4.html

Rasmussen, E. (2001). Picture imperfect: From Nurse Ratched to Hot Lips Houlihan, film/TV portrayals of nurses often transmit a warped image of real-life RN's. *NurseWeek.* Retrieved October 2, 2005, from http://www.nurseweek.com/news/features/01–05/picture.html

Sherman, G. (2000). *Nurses for a Healthier Tomorrow image campaign.* Unpublished manuscript prepared for Nurses for a Healthier Tomorrow, the American Association of Colleges of Nursing, Washington, DC.

Sochalski, J. (2002). Nursing shortage redux: Turning the corner on an enduring problem. *Health Affairs, 21*(5), 157–164.

Sports Illustrated. (2003, October 13). *99*(4), 94.

University of Portland School of Nursing. (2003). [Findings of male, guidance counselor, and student nurse focus groups]. Unpublished raw data and meeting proceedings.

Vincent, J. (Producer), & Roach, J. (Director). (2001). *Meet the parents* [Motion picture]. United States: Universal Studios.

Washington University School of Medicine. (2004). Men in nursing, occupational therapy and physical therapy. *Women in Health Sciences.* Retrieved October 2, 2005, from http://beckerexhibits.wustl.edu/mowihsp/stats/men.htm

Williams, C. (1983). *Image-making in nursing.* Kansas City, MO: American Nurses Association.

Williams, D. (2003). Looking for a few good men. *Minority Nurse.* Retrieved October 2, 2005, from http://www.minoritynurse.com/features/nurse_emp/05–03–02a.html

CHAPTER FIFTEEN

Men's Health: A Leadership Role for Men in Nursing

Demetrius J. Porche

INTRODUCTION

A silent crisis is affecting the health and well-being of men. Men are experiencing a disparity in morbidity and mortality as evidenced by men dying at a younger age than females. Without immediate action, this crisis will continue to threaten the health and well-being of men, their significant others, and their families, communities, and society. The men's health crisis has an impact beyond the male population, affecting women who lose their fathers, husbands, sons, and brothers to premature disease or death; affecting employers due to medical expenditures and loss of productive employees; and affecting state and federal governments due to the societal cost of premature morbidity and mortality. Men's health is an emerging and important area of research and practice within nursing (Porche & Willis, 2004). Men's health has not been defined in a clear and comprehensive manner. This chapter will explore the historical evolution of men's health, definitions of men's health, the need to focus on men's health issues, and nursing's proposed leadership role in men's health.

HISTORICAL EVOLUTION OF MEN'S HEALTH

The sociocultural model developed in the 1960s as a means of understanding health and illness challenged the biological determinism and reductionism of the traditional medical model. Rather than providing a medical model, this model emphasized culture, social conditions, emotions, environment, and personal beliefs as determinants in the morbidity and mortality of men (Sabo, 2000). Research focused on the gender stereotypes of the diagnosis and treatment of women. Men's health issues were not considered at this time. In the 1970s, men's health began to emerge in an exploratory fashion. Feminist theory and politics conceptualized men's health in relation to the premise that men's conformity to the masculine role produced health deficits.

Sex-role theory impacted the development of men's health in the 1980s. Scholars initiated dialogue regarding the study of men and masculinity with the assertion that masculinity was "potentially lethal" (Sabo, 2000). Sex-role theory was the predominant framework for research and influenced the examination of health differences in men and women based on how they perceived and experienced health and illness. Also in the 1980s, gay rights activists initiated activities to include more health promotion and health services for men. Gay identities and relationships became more transparent, prompting the integration of gay men's health issues into the discussions and debates regarding men's health.

Men, masculinity, and health were analyzed by critical feminists in the 1990s. Critical feminist scholars emphasized the power differences that were shaping relationships between men and women, women and women, and men and men. These scholars contended that gender identity and behavior not only occurred through socialization but was also cognitively constructed and best understood within the framework of the larger contextual institutional processes in which gender, masculinity, and health occurred (Courtenay, 2000; Sabo, 2000). Men's health scholars began to emerge in the 1990s. These scholars integrated race, ethnicity, social class, and sexual orientation into discussions regarding the contextual parameters in which gender impacted men's health processes and outcomes (Courtenay, 2000). During this time, male-specific and male-gender-prevalent illnesses such as testicular cancer, prostate cancer, alcohol abuse, suicide, violence, sports injury, and human immunodeficiency virus/acquired immune deficiency syndrome (HIV/AIDS) were emerging as men's health issues. During this time, the HIV/AIDS epidemic focused men's health issues on determinants of health such as unsafe sexual practices and drug use by injection.

Research in the period from the 1990s to the present has continued to identify the disparate trends in morbidity and mortality between men and women. Also, the identification of specific at-risk male populations with unique health risks and needs emerged. Men's health is currently being defined as an area of specialization that embraces a men's health paradigm with a wellness focus on the biologic/physiologic, psychological, social, environmental, developmental, and spiritual determinants of health (Porche & Willis, 2004; R. White, 2002).

MEN'S HEALTH DEFINED

Men's health has only in the last 10 years emerged as a significant health care movement (A. White, 2004). The men's health movement initially focused on male-specific illnesses involving anatomical differences between men and women. Currently, the men's health movement has evolved to extend beyond male-specific illnesses, but much confusion remains as to "What is men's health?" A challenge for the men's health movement is to reach a clear definition of and consensus on what constitutes men's health.

Multiple definitions have been proposed to clarify the area of men's health. Definitions of men's health vary dependent upon a country's paradigm. The Australian Men's Health Network defines men's health issues as conditions or diseases that are unique to men, more prevalent in men, or more serious among men, and for which the risk factors are different for men or for which different interventions are required for men (Fletcher, 1997). The Men's Health Forum of England describes a male health issue as one that arises from physiological, psychological, social, or environmental factors that have a specific impact on boys or men and/or where interventions are required to achieve health improvements in health and well-being at either the individual or the population level (Men's Health Forum, 2004; A. White, 2004).

In the United States, men's health has been defined as a holistic, comprehensive approach that addresses the physical, mental, emotional, social, and spiritual life-experiences and needs of men throughout their life span in order to promote health (Porche & Willis, 2004). What constitutes men's health is also defined through definitions of men's health studies. Sabo (2000) defines men's health studies as a systematic analysis of men's health and illness that considers gender and gender health equity in the theoretical context.

Regardless of the definition selected to describe the parameters of men's health, the essential defining elements of men's health are (a) conditions unique to and prevalent in men; (b) a holistic approach that includes the biologic/physiologic, psychological, social, environmental, developmental, and spiritual needs of men; and (c) interventions that are uniquely based on the determinants of conditions specific to and prevalent in men. It is imperative to note that men's health expands beyond the biological paradigm into relevance as a social issue (R. White, 2002). Men's health is intricately related to masculinity. Debates and discussions regarding men's health should include masculinity as a central issue.

OVERVIEW OF THE DETERMINANTS
OF MEN'S HEALTH

The disparities that exist between men and women provide a substantive rationale for the relevance of men's health. The life expectancy of men in the United States is about six years less than that of women (Meyer, 2003); males 15 to 19 years of age are 2.5 times more likely to die of an unintentional injury than women and five times more likely to die of homicide or suicide; and infant males are more likely to die in their first year of life than infant females (Williams, 2003). These morbidity and mortality statistics reveal the tip of the iceberg of the disparity that exists in male health from infancy to older adulthood.

Men's morbidity and mortality are impacted by determinants such as social and societal factors. Male marginality (Willis & Porche, 2004), occupational status, working conditions and their related stressors, personal health practices, and health care service utilization (Williams, 2003) represent social, behavioral, and societal determinants of health. For example, behavioral determinants of men's health include the fact that men are more likely to smoke cigarettes and consume five or more alcoholic drinks in a single day. In addition, evidence suggests that men experience higher levels of employment-related stress. Men have fewer preventive health care visits, visit a doctor less frequently, and have lower levels of medical treatment adherence than women (Williams, 2003). Other determinants of men's health focus on the conceptualization of male gender.

Men's gender identity is not constructed solely within the context of men's lives but is constructed in a perceived relationship with respect to women within a cultural context (Sabo, 2000). The gender-identity constructions of masculinity and femininity occur with respect to hegemonic masculinity and emphasized femininity (Connell, 1987). Hegemonic masculinity accentuates male dominance over women, physical strength, proneness to violence, emotional inexpressiveness, and competitiveness (Sabo, 2000). Emphasized femininity accentuates the cultural beliefs that women are sociable, fragile, passive, compliant with men's desires, and sexually receptive (Sabo, 2000). Conformity to these hegemonic masculinities by men can pose health risks. Men are more likely to engage in high-risk behaviors or activities as a means to prove or integrate the expected hegemonic perspective of masculinity. Research has identified the fact that masculine ideology has been associated with school suspension, drinking and the use of illicit drugs, arrest by police, and polygamous and unsafe sexual activity (Sabo, 2000). These health determinants pose significant health risks to men and deserve attention in the effort to improve men's health. The impact of these determinants on the state of men's health accentuates the need for an area of specialization focusing on men's health.

In addition to these determinants, the prevalence of programs that do not embrace men's particular needs in relation to services and access, a lack of awareness, poor health education, a paucity of male-specific health programs and health care systems, and a paucity of male-gender-specific health research all contribute to the deteriorating state of men's health (Meyer, 2003; Porche & Willis, 2004). Existing health care delivery systems frequently fail to integrate men's particular health needs, experiences, and concerns (Baker, 2001). A men's health movement is urgently needed to coordinate the fragmented men's health initiatives, develop male-specific health promotion and disease prevention programs, promote gender-specific research efforts, and coordinate men's health outreach and community awareness campaigns (Porche & Willis, 2004). Nursing has a great opportunity to assume a leadership role in facilitating the evolution and development of a men's health specialty.

NURSING'S LEADERSHIP ROLE IN MEN'S HEALTH

Nursing has been slow to respond to men's health as a defined area of specialization. However, nursing has taken the leadership in calling the profession to action to consider a specific advanced-practice role in men's health at least three times in the published literature (Bozett & Forrester, 1989; Forrester, 2000; Porche & Willis, 2004). Specialized men's health practitioners are critical to ensuring the future of men's health. These practitioners would have the potential to develop the nursing knowledge base on men's health as a means of decreasing the gender disparity and improving the quality of men's lives.

Nursing, as a discipline that is highly respected by the public, has an opportunity to provide future directions and mobilize communities and societies. Men's health should not be permitted to become a public health crisis. The future of men's health is dependent upon nursing strategies targeting men, and upon health care professionals and policymakers. Primarily, men should take responsibility for their own health; however, health care practitioners should be aware of and proactively manage conditions impacting men's health. Policymakers must advocate for policy actions that reduce the gender health disparities men experience (Kirby, 2004). Policymakers have the ability to ensure that there are adequate fiscal resources to promote a men's health agenda with the priority of supporting the development of male-specific programs and research. *Men in nursing have a unique opportunity to impact men's health as members of the male population, as members of the nursing profession, and as political activists.*

As health educators, nurses have an opportunity to teach parents about the impact of masculine socialization upon boys and men's health outcomes throughout their lives. Nurses are responsible for ensuring that health literature and health education include male-specific topics such as male breast cancer, testicular cancer, and prostate cancer. There should be a conscientious effort to ensure that health literature and health education encompass the full spectrum of men's health issues.

Nurses should have a high index of awareness and sensitivity regarding men's health issues and should develop health care systems that integrate men's health services. Men do not typically access the health care system. Therefore, men in nursing, with their knowledge of male behavior, should advocate for the development of innovative health care systems that ensure access to and utilization of health care services. Health care services developed specifically for men should be comprehensive in nature, focusing on all aspects of male health issues. For example, health care services should be developed to provide care for men who are perpetrators of violence but should also focus on men as victims of violence, inclusive of male sexual assault.

Nursing education has an opportunity to assume a leadership role in defining the scope of practice in men's health as a means to decrease the gender disparity in morbidity and mortality. Men's health content should be integrated into nursing curricula at the associate's, bachelor's, master's, and doctoral levels. Nursing has an opportunity to develop an advanced-practice role in men's health for a nurse practitioner with the knowledge, skills, and scope of practice to address men's health from an integrated biomedical and nursing model. The biomedical model would focus on delineating pathological findings, differential medical diagnosis, and prescription of treatments targeting the medical diagnosis (Forrester, 2000). The nursing model would emphasize holistic, comprehensive care focusing on health promotion, disease prevention, and nursing interventions within a population-based framework (Porche & Willis, 2004). In addition, the nursing model would embrace a wellness framework with a holistic approach that incorporates at least three types of nursing interventions: the biological determinants of health and well-being, the structure of gender relations, and the social differences and inequalities within the male population (R. White, 2002). Proposed content for a men's health nurse-practitioner curriculum is outlined in Table 15.1. A comprehensive primary-care, men's health nurse-practitioner curriculum should provide information in the domains of physiological, psychological, and sociocultural variables (Bozett & Forrester, 1989), health policy, case management, and program planning. Forrester (2000) proposes that a men's health nurse-practitioner curriculum should embrace essential wellness dimensions of well-being that are inclusive of social, physical, occupational, intellectual, emotional, and spiritual wellness.

There is a paucity of nursing research on men's health. A common misunderstanding is that most of the research that has been conducted has been on men's health. This inaccuracy is a result of a misunderstanding as to what constitutes men's health. Men have historically been

TABLE 15.1   Recommendations for Men's Health Nurse-Practitioner Curriculum Content

- Dynamic relationship between environment, lifestyle, and biology
- Male growth and development—biologic, psychologic, and sociocultural
- Lifestyle and transitions—career issues, relationship changes, age-specific changes
- Men's health promotion and disease prevention
- Healthy aging
- Acute and chronic illnesses affecting men (including mental and physical illness) as observed in population-based morbidity and mortality data
- Occupational health issues
- Gender and sexual orientation specific health promotion, disease prevention, and illness management
- Health policy and political processes
- Men's health program planning and development
- Masculine role socialization and its impact on men's health (primary and secondary socialization)
- Violence and incarceration
- Males as sexual assault victims
- Parenting/fathering
- Relationships, marriage, and divorce
- Genetic counseling
- Sexual health and counseling
- Changing identities
- Male reproductive conditions
- Male responsibility in family planning
- Anger management, conflict resolution and emotional expression
- Minority men's health issues
- Gay and bisexual health issues
- Men in the family
- Men and spirituality and religion
- Conduct and dissemination of men's health nursing research

the primary subjects in research, but men have not been the subject of research (White & Johnson, 1998). Nurses need to initiate and develop programs of nursing research on men's health. Programs of nursing research on men's health should focus on the Healthy People 2010 goals and objectives, with the intent of reducing the health disparities resulting from the gender gap.

SUMMARY

Men are experiencing a great disparity in health compared with women, as evidenced in the gender gap in morbidity and mortality statistics. There is a critical lack of health care programs and systems specifically targeting the unique men's health issues that men experience. Nurses, specifically men in nursing, have the opportunity to assume a leadership role in the integration of men's health content in curricula. Additionally, a men's health nurse-practitioner role would promote evidence-based men's health practice and expand the knowledge base on effective nursing interventions in order to impact the quality of men's lives. Nurses, including men in nursing, as members of the most trusted of health care disciplines, should capitalize on their reputation with the public to promote quality male health programs and a men's health agenda.

REFERENCES

Baker, P. (2001). The state of men's health. *Men's Health Journal, 1*(1), 6–8.

Bozett, F. W., & Forrester, D. A. (1989). A proposal for a men's health nurse practitioner. *Image: Journal of Nursing Scholarship, 21*(3), 158–161.

Connell, R. W. (1987). *Gender and power.* Stanford, CA: Stanford University Press.

Courtenay, W. (2000). Constructions of masculinity and their influence on men's well-being. *Social Science and Medicine, 50*(10), 1385–1401.

Fletcher, R. (1997). *Report on men's health services.* Newcastle, England: University of Newcastle.

Forrester, D. A. (2000). Revisiting the men's health curriculum. In *Understanding cultural diversity: Culture, curriculum, and community in nursing* (pp. 169–175). Sudbury, MA: Jones and Bartlett Publishers, Inc.

Kirby, M. (2004). Erectile dysfunction: A model for men's health. *Journal of Men's Health and Gender, 1*(2–3), 255–258.

Men's Health Forum. (2004). *Getting it sorted.* London: Author.

Meyer, J. A. (2003). Improving men's health: Developing a long-term strategy. *American Journal of Public Health, 93*(5), 709–711.

Porche, D. J., & Willis, D. G. (2004). Nursing and the men's health movement: Considerations for the 21st century. *Nursing Clinics of North America, 39*(2), 251–258.

Sabo, D. (2000). Men's health studies: Origins and trends. *Journal of American College Health, 49*(3), 133–142.

White, A. (2004). Men's health: The challenges ahead. *Journal of Men's Health and Gender,* *1*(4), 296–299.

White, A., & Johnson, M. (1998). The complexities of nursing research with men. *International Journal of Nursing Studies, 35*(1–2), 41–48.

White, R. (2002). Social and political aspects of men's health. *Health: An Interdisciplinary Journal for the Social Study of Health, Illness, and Medicine, 6*(3), 267–285.

Williams, D. R. (2003). The health of men: Structured inequalities and opportunities. *American Journal of Public Health, 93*(5), 724–731.

Willis, D. G., & Porche, D. J. (2004). Male battering of intimate partners: Theoretical underpinnings, intervention approaches, and implications. *Nursing Clinics of North America, 39*(2), 271–282.

Epilogue

Russell E. Tranbarger

As a small child I received a doctor's kit, and after listening to my dad's chest with the toy stethoscope, I solemnly notified him that he was not expected to live through the night. That is one of the childhood events that was repeated many times over the years and seemed to form my desire to become a physician. During the first year of college it became apparent to me that I could not afford college. John Garde, a friend of mine from the same small farming community in Illinois, told me that if I became a nurse I could then become a nurse anesthetist and work my way through medical school. That seemed to make sense to me, and so I naïvely began to apply for admission to schools of nursing. Some schools simply did not respond to my inquiries. Some schools informed me that nursing was for women and they would not accept me or any man into their program. Fortunately John had also told me about the Alexian Brothers Hospital School of Nursing in Chicago where he was enrolled.

I applied and was accepted by the Alexian Brothers and began my nursing education along with 54 other men ranging from 17 to 35 years of age. By this time, I had developed sensitivity to how others reacted to the fact that I was in nursing school. A female cousin of mine in the third grade got into a fight with a classmate who insisted that since I was a man I could not be in nursing school but surely must be in medical school. Thus, I told most people that I was attending DePaul University in Chicago, technically correct since we took our non-nursing sciences there. It was perhaps six months before I had the courage to tell close friends that I was actually enrolled in nursing school. At the completion of the first semester, or the preclinical phase, we received our blue diamond pin in a formal ceremony before an audience of family and friends. By this point I understood that nursing was what I wanted to do for the rest of

my life and neither nurse anesthesia or medicine held any attraction for
me.

Thanks to the Alexian Brothers and the men in nursing during my
student days, I developed a strong belief that nursing was a valid profession for both men and women. I benefited from the many role models I
had, as well as both female and male mentors who guided me into professional practice. It was as though we were in a bubble or cocoon and men
in nursing were as ordinary as food, light, or air. What mattered most
was whether we were proficient and accurate in our nursing practice!

Graduation and entry into the larger world of nursing brought me
to understand Marlene Kramer's culture-conflict concepts before I had
ever heard of her or her concepts! I was the first man hired as a nurse at
a large children's hospital in Chicago. Many of the nurses signed a peti-
tion objecting to my employment, even though they had never met me.
Nevertheless, I was hired anyway, and the children who were my patients
warmly welcomed me. My arrival was during the last stages of the post-
polio era, and many boys between the ages of 3 and 18 were patients
there for lengthy periods of time. I remember that we watched the Miss
America Pageant in the older boys' ward, even though it was shown after the televisions were supposed to be turned off. I arranged for Friday
evenings to be "date nights" for the patients. The girls washed their hair
and put on makeup, while the boys talked with each other about what
they planned to discuss with the girls. I would then place the stretcher of
a girl next to the stretcher of the boy who was her date that night in a
corner of the ward.

During my career, I continued to work to make gender unimportant
in nursing but continued to discover that others wanted to continue to
make gender essential to practice. In my experience, patients cared little
about my gender but a great deal about how I treated them. If I was quick
to help them and effective in my care for them, then the fact that I was a
man was only a momentary distraction. I continued to be amazed at the
reaction of nurses and hospital administrators to the issue of men in nursing. More than one hospital administrator told me he would never hire
a man in any capacity, because only women could be good nurses. Some
eventually changed their minds after they had the experience of working
with a man in nursing.

Perhaps my most challenging experience came when I applied for
graduate school. I was accepted and enrolled for my first semester of
graduate studies. I was called to my faculty advisor's office for a counseling session. She advised me that no man had ever passed her course. She
informed me that men who entered nursing, in her opinion, were inadequate men and became incompetent nurses. She then said she saw no
reason why my experience would be any different from that of the other

men who had previously tried to graduate from the program. She told me that if I resigned from the university, perhaps another program would accept me. If I insisted on remaining here I would fail her course, the university would terminate me, and no other university would ever accept me again. She gave me 24 hours to decide to resign and told me to leave her office. After a period of reflection, some depression, and perhaps a libation or two, I decided to force her to fail me. In the end, I received a good grade from her. She repeatedly told me that I was different from the other men in nursing she had known, a response that members of minority groups hear often. Somehow, I was either more competent than previous men students, or was it that she felt I was less of a male? Whatever the cause, she turned into a supporter of mine, but I must admit that I never developed much respect for her!

I would like to think that trivial issues of gender are behind us in nursing today. Yet the discussion forum hosted by the American Assembly for Men in Nursing seems to indicate that men entering nursing today face many of the same problems, attitudes, and discrimination as in the past. It may be more subtle today. However, I genuinely believe the public's perception is greatly different from that of our female nurse colleagues. The public has moved far beyond the nursing profession in accepting men as nurses.

I hope that by developing this book we will have documented a history of nursing that has included men from history far earlier than today's nurses ever imagined. I hope we will give comfort to our male colleagues who read the stories of the success that men in nursing have achieved. I hope we will silence our enemies who for reasons of jealousy or other reasons try to keep men from becoming nurses or try to prevent them from enjoying the free and full practice of their skills. I strongly believe that a more diverse profession of nursing will be more caring of its diverse client population, more supportive of colleagues, and even more respected by the public. Men and women in nursing have a rich history and a vibrant future together!

R. E. T.

Index